After Breast Cancer

A Recovery Handbook

After Breast Cancer

A Recovery Handbook

A guide for moving forward and navigating your way
through post-treatment life after breast cancer

SARA LIYANAGE

sheldon PRESS

First published in Great Britain by Sheldon Press in 2023
An imprint of John Murray Press
A division of Hodder & Stoughton Ltd,
An Hachette UK company

1

This book is for information or educational purposes only and is not intended to act as a substitute for medical advice or treatment. Any person with a condition requiring medical attention should consult a qualified medical practitioner or suitable therapist.

A CIP catalogue record for this title is available from the British Library

Trade Paperback ISBN 9781399808019
eBook ISBN 9781399808026

Typeset by KnowledgeWorks Global Ltd.

Printed and bound in Great Britain by Clays Ltd, Elcograf S.p.A.

John Murray Press policy is to use papers that are natural, renewable and recyclable products and made from wood grown in sustainable forests. The logging and manufacturing processes are expected to conform to the environmental regulations of the country of origin.

John Murray Press
Carmelite House
50 Victoria Embankment
London EC4Y 0DZ

www.sheldonpress.co.uk

Acknowledgements

This book is a collaboration effort and without the input of my contributors – interviewees and experts – there wouldn't be a book. I would like to say a huge thank you to all the women who spoke to me about their experience of life after breast cancer treatment: Amy Gates, Carly Moosah, Cathy Murphy, Emily Jones, Fi Donnison, Gabi Holbrook, Gloria Nelson, Iyna Butt, Jo Hammond, Jo Long, Julie Wimberly, Juliet Fitzpatrick, Kate Ware, Kathryn Hulland, Laura Dampney, Leanne Pero, Lindsey Cave, Mary Perry, Melissa Golding, Molly Slominski, Natasha Whelehan, Nevo Burrell, Nina Lopes, Rachel Bayliss, Rachel Le Mesurier, Ruth Lavendar, Sara Green, Tasha Horner, Toni-Ann La-Crette and Vicky Tarran. I am so grateful to every single one of these women who opened up and talked to me at length about the challenges and difficulties they have faced since completing their treatment. Their honest – and often emotional – accounts are what have shaped this book from the outset.

I would also like to say an equally huge thank you to the group of experts who provided their professional insight and advice for each of the chapters: Allie Morgan, Anne Crook, Barbara Babcock, Dr Jane Clark, Lyndel Moore and Dr Sophie McGrath. I spent many hours – often on multiple occasions – talking to this team of experts and I've had numerous e-mail exchanges with each of them. I am immensely grateful to them for their time, patience, understanding and constant support.

I would also like to thank everyone who has supported me during the process of putting this book together, by reading and sense checking drafts and allowing me to run ideas past them.

Thank you to the Future Dreams Breast Cancer Charity for their constant – amazing – support with this project.

And importantly, a very big thank you to Victoria and the team at Sheldon Press for believing in this book, taking it – and me – on, and creating something that will help those people who are finishing their breast cancer treatment and struggling with navigating their way forward.

Contents

Introduction

Life after breast cancer

Hello and welcome to *After Breast Cancer: A Recovery Handbook*. The sequel – of sorts – to my first book, *Ticking Off Breast Cancer*. This book is for anyone who has finished treatment for cancer. Whilst it's focused on issues arising after breast cancer treatment, it's equally applicable to anyone who's had any type of cancer. This book is:

- a companion for those of you who're in the post-treatment period and feeling like you're the only one who's going through a tough time
- an aide for those of you who are confused about how you're feeling and are trying to make sense of what's going on
- for anyone who has finished treatment for cancer – whether last week, last month or years ago
- a guide for those around you, your family and friends, to understand what you're going through.

The book focuses on the challenges faced by someone after breast cancer, but it will also provide advice and insight to anyone who has finished cancer treatment – whether breast cancer or another type of cancer.

Some statistics to start us off

Before I tell you more about this book, I'd like to mention some statistics in order to put into context, why there is a need for a book such as this. Contrary to what you might have thought before you had cancer, a lot of people who are diagnosed with cancer do not go on to die from it. Survival rates differ greatly between types of cancer, depending on the ease/difficulty in diagnosing and treating the different types of cancer, but looking at cancer patients as a group, a significant proportion of people who are diagnosed with cancer in the UK, will survive for five, ten or even more years after treatment.

According to Cancer Research UK,[1] 50 per cent of all people diagnosed with cancer in England and Wales will survive for at least ten years. In fact, Cancer Research UK's statistics show that 78 per cent of all women diagnosed with breast cancer in England and Wales will survive at least ten years. Thanks to modern advances in cancer medicine, more and more people are having their cancer successfully removed and are living beyond cancer.

All this is amazing, fantastic and wonderful. It truly is. However, despite more people having successful treatment and living beyond cancer, the impact of having had a cancer diagnosis and having gone through treatment is still enormously significant for them. Every one of these people has sat in a plastic chair somewhere deep within the maze of a hospital and heard the words, *you've got cancer.* They've lived through a hellish time of scans, appointments, blood tests, surgery, chemotherapy, radiotherapy and quite possibly a raft of other treatments. Some of these people may need to continue to take medication to help prevent the cancer from returning and some will be undergoing some form of regular medical review, for example annual mammograms for people who've had breast cancer. Even though their treatment has been successful, these people will all have been impacted – to differing extents – on a physical, emotional and mental level by the fact that they have had cancer.

Everyone is different

The impact of having had cancer and going through cancer treatment affects people in different ways. I tend to think of the spectrum of impact as a scale: on one hand there are those for whom having had cancer causes minimal or no emotional impact and only a short period of physical side-effects. Once they've got over any side-effects, they quickly return to their pre-cancer life as if cancer had not happened.

On the other hand, there are those people for whom the impact of having had cancer will never go and they are affected by it for the rest of their lives whether on a physical, emotional and/or mental level. It's all-consuming and affects many aspects of daily life.

And then you have everyone else – the majority of people – who are somewhere in between these two extremes. People for whom having had a cancer diagnosis causes some emotional and mental health challenges together with some physical issues that can hang around for a period of time after the end of treatment. People for whom finishing cancer treat-ment isn't quite the end of their cancer experience that they'd hoped for, but for whom it's just the start of a new – somewhat difficult – chapter in their lives. Yes, it's true that there is a minority group for whom nothing is changed by cancer – but they're not reading this book. You're reading this book because something has changed. You will fall somewhere between these two extremes.

What next?

When you get to the end of cancer treatment and you realize that it's not a simple case of picking up life where you left off before you were diagnosed with cancer, it can invoke a huge range of emotions from frustration to anger to grief to loss. In fact, reaching the end of treatment and realizing that there's a lot more to 'moving on' than you might have thought can be pretty scary. You might feel like you're the only one struggling with this stage; that nobody understands how you're feeling and you're unsure where to turn to for help.

This is where this book comes in. It's a book for all of you who've finished treatment and realized that moving on with your life isn't going to be quite as straightforward as you'd expected – or hoped.

What is this book about?

This book is a heads up of what to expect when the treatment ends. It explores some of the challenges that you may face as you embark on – and move through – this stage of recovery, and even challenges that might remain after weeks, months or years. Not everyone will experience all of them, and there may be some challenges not covered by this book. But the aims of this book are to:

- share some personal anecdotes of other people's experiences so that you know you're not alone in how you're feeling;
- explain, with the help of some experts, that the emotions and feelings that you're experiencing are normal at this stage of treatment;
- provide you with some practical advice, coping mechanisms and tools to start processing what you're going through.

This book doesn't pretend to answer all the questions or deal with all the issues experienced by everyone. It's a starting point from which to do your own research, talk to people who can help you and set your own agenda for recovery. It recognizes that everyone's experience is different but it addresses the common issues felt by people who've had cancer.

How to use this book

I recommend that you read the book in its entirety, however if you've only recently completed your cancer treatment you might find it slightly overwhelming to immediately read this book from cover to cover. Instead, it might help to take a chapter at a time. However, it's important to be aware that sometimes it can be hard to address a single challenge on its own and sometimes addressing one thing might bring up other feelings that you haven't previously addressed.

Whilst each chapter deals with a different challenge, in reality each challenge is often interconnected and linked to the others. It's important to look at the whole picture of what you're going through and keep that in mind as you move forward with your recovery.

Each chapter includes some suggested exercises or action points that will help you deal with the challenge covered in that chapter. Whilst working through the exercises in one chapter, you might find that these bring up some other feelings. Let me give you an example. Imagine you are feeling guilty for being a burden on your elderly parents during your cancer treatment. You'll read the chapter on guilt and then start to work on the exercises described in that chapter. This might make you realize that actually your feelings of guilt relate to feelings of vulnerability and a loss of control. And as you start to sit with these feelings, you might notice that they stem from your fear of a cancer recurrence. And when you start to think about recurrence you notice your heart beats faster and your palms get all sweaty. You lose focus on what you're doing and you might feel so overwhelmed that you decide to put this book down and get a glass – or three – of wine to try to relax. As you can see, just by thinking about the guilt you've been feeling, you've strayed into other complex feelings of vulnerability, loss, lack of control, fear of recurrence and anxiety. And this can feel overwhelming. But don't panic and don't give up. Maybe take a break, have a cup of tea, do some exercise, sit in the garden, go for a walk or bake some – healthy – cookies. Then, a little later in the day or in a few days' time – you can come back to the exercises refreshed and ready to work on them.

At the end of each chapter is a checklist recapping the key points covered in the chapter so you can refer back to the checklists as and when you need a reminder of the insights and advice given on a particular issue. Also at the end of each chapter is a page for your notes. You can write notes about how you relate to the insight given in the chapter; you can write about how you feel after reading that chapter; you can write about your experience relevant to the issues raised in the chapter; and you can write notes about how you plan to address any issues that come up after reading the chapter.

Towards the back of the book is the Toolkit. The Toolkit is full of practical advice and strategies for coping with and dealing with the challenges you face as you move through this stage of recovery, as discussed and suggested in each of the chapters. You'll find breathing exercises; mindfulness exercises; affirmations; advice on journalling and writing including writing prompts and writing a gratitude journal; and tips for creating a healthy bedtime routine.

There are plenty of resources listed in the Useful Resources section at the back of the book: places where you'll find help and support for dealing with the issues you face at the end of cancer treatment.

This isn't a medical reference book. It's worth noting that whilst there is some expert and professional advice in each chapter, this book is intended to be your starting point from which you can then move forward with your recovery – perhaps by using some of the tools in the Toolkit but also perhaps by recognizing where you might need some professional help.

Reaching the end of treatment and moving forward with your life is far more complex than many people expect and it's perfectly normal to feel scared and confused rather than elated. In fact, even just sitting with uncomfortable thoughts can be incredibly tricky. So always remember, if you're struggling, it's important to seek professional help: talk to your doctor, your oncologist, oncology nursing team, psychologist or counsellor.

Recovering from cancer treatment doesn't have a time limit. Cancer can send out ripples long after treatment has ended so you might be reading this book because you are still experiencing some of these challenges at some point down the line after treatment – months or even years. That's fine. This book is for you too.

Who am I?

You might be wondering who I am and why I'm writing a book about life after cancer. Well, I was diagnosed with primary breast cancer in 2016 at the age of 42. I went through surgery, chemotherapy, radiotherapy and targeted biological therapy (Herceptin). I'm still on hormone therapy (Tamoxifen) and I expect to continue to take this for a total of ten years. After my treatment I set up a website to support people going through breast cancer treatment and beyond – www.tickingoffbreastcancer.com. In 2019, my first book was published, *Ticking Off Breast Cancer*, which is part memoir and part self-help giving a heads-up of what to expect from breast cancer treatment together with plenty of practical advice (and checklists) for getting through the treatment. In 2021 I joined the Future Dreams Breast Cancer Charity family to run the support section of their website. And I'm also a writer, speaker and general advocate on the topic of cancer.

Why did I write this book?

Whilst going through my breast cancer treatment I would dream of getting to the end of radiotherapy, having a big party to celebrate, taking a few weeks to properly recuperate and then hopping back onto the conveyor belt of normal life where I'd left off the day I'd been diagnosed. I honestly thought that with a few extra weeks off work to build up my strength, I'd be back in the saddle of normal life within a month of the end of treatment.

But when it came to it, that's certainly not what happened. For a while I couldn't quite understand why life didn't go straight back to the way it had been before cancer. I thought there was something wrong with me ... the intense fatigue, the non-stop crying, the panic attacks, the inability to sleep, the fear of recurrence, the heightened anxiety, the guilt, the loss of confidence and the fear of leaving the house. This wasn't meant to be happening. I was meant to feel elated and relieved. I hadn't been prepared for any of this and I didn't know how to cope with it all.

But now, five years down the line, I know that everything that I went through was 100 per cent normal and, in fact, the vast majority of cancer patients experience most, if not all, of the difficulties I was experiencing. I also realized that, in fact, there are plenty of challenges that I didn't personally experience but which other people were experiencing. We're all different and there are a lot of challenges being faced by people as they try to move forward with their lives after cancer treatment. Not everyone experiences everything, but there are certainly some areas of commonality.

During my recovery and in my work within the breast cancer community over the past few years, it struck me that whilst we're all facing challenges to differing extents, the support for these challenges is mixed depending on where you live, the hospital at which you had your treatment and the availability of local support. Support is out there: sometimes we're informed about it by our medical team, but sometimes we're not. It's often down to us to find it but this all relies upon us knowing what to look for, where to look for it and how to access it. Which can be easier said than done.

So, I've created this book for anyone getting to the end of treatment and not knowing which way to turn. It's really a guide. A guide to addressing the challenges faced after cancer treatment – specifically breast cancer treatment. It will help you identify what you're going through; show that you're certainly not alone in experiencing these challenges; help you understand why you're going through them; and give you some advice for dealing with them.

The book's credentials

I've had breast cancer. I'm moving on and I've experienced many of the challenges covered in this book. But this book isn't about me. Part of running a breast cancer support website over the past few years has involved talking to lots of people about this stage of cancer recovery. I've talked to lots of people who've been through cancer. I've talked to people who finished treatment last week and to people who finished treatment over ten years ago, plus plenty of people in the middle. As part of my specific research for this book I interviewed over thirty women[2] of all ages and backgrounds, about their experiences after completing primary breast cancer and moving forward with their lives.

These women[3] are all at different stages of post-treatment with some only just having completed their treatment and others having finished treatment a number of years ago. They had different types of breast cancer, different treatment plans at different hospitals, different side-effects and have experienced (or are still experiencing) different challenges. But there are a lot of commonalities across their experiences and these are the challenges I've included in this book: anxiety, losing a safety net of treatment, fear of recurrence, trauma, flashbacks, loss, grief, loneliness, loss of confidence, loss of trust, guilt, the impact upon the rest of the family and lingering physical challenges. In this book you will find personal anecdotes from these women and reading about their experiences will remind you that you are certainly not alone in what you're going through.

Given that I'm not an expert at moving on with life after cancer – I'm not a psychologist or a counsellor or medically trained in any way – all the expert and professional advice in this book comes from real experts and professionals. Research for the book involved talking to a range of professionals,[4] including an oncologist, an oncology nurse, a clinical psychologist, a psycho-oncology counsellor, a confidence coach and a life coach: all of whom are well placed to give insight and advice on coping with the hurdles you may face as you try to move on from cancer. The advice and insight contained in this book comes from them.

I hope that you'll find encouragement, advice, hope and a little bit of hand-holding in the pages of this book.

Wishing you all the very best, with much love,
Sara x

Life doesn't come with an instruction manual

Someone once told me that life is like a complicated model – for which you have no instruction manual – constructed out of thousands of little Lego bricks. You know the little building bricks of varying colours, shapes and sizes that can be bought in packs to build all sorts of amazing structures from well-known landmarks to famous fictional spaceships and even entire towns? Well, imagine this … for as long as you can remember, you've been building your life model from these little bricks. It's in pretty good shape. There might be a couple of parts stuck together with glue and tape and some parts may look a little different to how you'd planned when you started out building the model, but on the whole it's looking good. You've got it on display up on the sideboard where you add to it and change it from time to time, following the pattern of your life.

But then, one day, cancer comes along and knocks your model off the sideboard causing it to shatter back into all those little individual bricks. For a while cancer takes up a lot of your time and attention as you go through treatment, so you can't do anything about the shattered model and all the little bricks that are strewn across the room.

Then, cancer treatment comes to an end and it's time to pick up all those little bricks and rebuild your life model. There's no instruction manual and so you have to work out how to rebuild it. In doing so, you soon realize that the process of rebuilding your model is actually quite complicated. You can't quite remember how some of the bricks fit together, some of the bricks are now missing and some of the bricks don't fit back together like they used to.

As you struggle to rebuild your model, you notice that you're not building the same model as before, yes there are some similar parts and some of the old parts are still there, but this version of your model is looking quite different to the old model – in fact you hardly even recognize parts of it.

Some parts of this new version of your model are particularly tricky to construct and you need help, but it's okay because there's actually a line of people queuing up to help you: family, friends, colleagues, neighbours, new friends you've made during cancer treatment, your oncologist, other members of the medical team from your hospital and maybe a counsellor or therapist. Some of them arrive with little bricks to slot into the new version of the model and some of them bring the glue or sticky tape to help keep the model together.

Gradually, with some hard work on your part, a few ups and downs along the way and plenty of tears, you manage to rebuild your model out of the thousands of shattered pieces. Some of you end up with models that look similar to the old version, whilst others of you create completely different models from those you had before cancer. Your model will inevitably alter over time, as you move forward in your life: it will take some hits, lose some bricks, gain some bricks and quite possibly need more glue and tape. But something is certain, even if it's a bit wobbly in places, there won't be a single day when you're not thankful for your model.

1

At the end of treatment

Facing physical, emotional and mental challenges after cancer treatment

'Cancer affects your body, but it also messes with your emotions and feelings. I'm still learning that sadness, guilt, fear, and anxiety are all normal. It's like a grieving process and I'm learning to cope with the changes in my life. I think it's important not to ignore these feelings but to talk about them and share them with others'.

Amy

So, your cancer treatment has ended. You've successfully completed weeks, months, possibly years of medical treatment for cancer, and finally your medical team has sent you on your way. Hooray!

To mark the end of treatment, you might have rung the 'end of treatment bell'. You know, those bells on the wall of the chemo ward that get rung when someone finishes treatment while their family and the nurses stand around clapping and taking photos. You might have taken cakes to the hospital to mark the last treatment and to thank the nurses. Your family and friends may have held a celebratory party for you. You might even have been on an amazing holiday with your loved ones or your fantastic tribe of supporters who've been there by your side since the day you found out that you had cancer. Or you might not have marked the end of treatment in any way other than with a nice hot drink and a bar of your favourite chocolate in front of the telly.

However you choose to mark the end of treatment, there is no doubt that this is a major milestone: it's a point at which you can let out the breath you've been holding in since you were told you had cancer. You can unhunch your shoulders, relax your jaw and breathe a huge sigh of relief because, of course, there's an enormous relief that treatment is over and that you no longer have to undergo those horrible chemo infusions, have radiation administered to part of your body or have needles regularly pushed into your veins for blood tests, cannulas and injections.

After all, cancer treatment is undoubtedly unpleasant and it will never be top of anyone's list of ways to spend their time.

Not only is having treatment for cancer highly unpleasant, it's also incredibly exhausting: travelling to hospital every day or every week is tiring; having chemo, immunotherapy or radiotherapy is tiring; coping with side-effects is tiring; and allowing your body to recover and rejuvenate is tiring. It is, quite honestly, tiring being tired.

In addition to not having to undergo actual treatment any longer, it's also a relief not to have to visit the hospital quite as frequently. During treatment, some of you will have been at the hospital every day whilst others will have been less frequently – perhaps weekly or every few weeks. No matter how frequently you visited, it's unlikely that you ever got used to, or felt completely comfortable with, the antiseptic smell and sterile atmosphere of a hospital. It's a place where ill people go. And nobody wants to be ill.

With the end of treatment there may also be relief that the immediate side-effects of treatment are easing – maybe less nausea, maybe fewer headaches and maybe it's easier to sleep. Not having day-to-day life dictated by hospital appointments will also be a relief and perhaps there will be time for the more important things in life, like seeing family, spending time with your children, socializing with friends and getting back to work.

So, the fact that you don't need to keep going to the hospital to be prodded and poked is surely a good thing, isn't it? Yes, it's a huge relief to no longer have to go to hospital to have treatment, but, in reality, it's common for this relief at finishing cancer treatment to be countered by a number of challenges.

A myriad of challenges

Being faced with a myriad of physical, emotional and mental challenges at the end of treatment, might come as a bit of a surprise to some of you. Perhaps even an outright shock. As you went through treatment, the focus was most likely – and rightly – on getting rid of the cancer. Very little consideration is usually given to what will happen once treatment comes to an end and when it comes, there is often a distinct difference between how you expect to feel versus how you actually feel.

It's quite possible that it's only now – at this point after treatment – that you fully recognize the enormity of what you've just been through. And with this realization comes an influx of physical, emotional and mental challenges. In fact, in almost every chapter of this book you will read that part of the reason you're only now experiencing these challenges is because it's only now that treatment is over – and you're off the treatment conveyor belt – that your brain has the space to start thinking about, and to process, what you've been through and what you're currently going through.

Emotions and feelings

Some of the normal emotions and feelings that you might experience at this stage include:

- a shock realization at what you've just been through
- fear at losing the safety net of hospital contact and treatment coupled with uncertainty and unease about what happens now: you may feel lost with no regular reassurance from your hospital team
- a lack of direction or purpose now that the busy period of going to hospital is over and you have more time on your hands
- loneliness because your friends and family may not understand how you're feeling – they might expect you to be 'back to normal' whilst in fact you may feel far from normal
- conflict with your partner/spouse because they may think that you should be getting over cancer and bouncing back, whilst in reality you might still be feeling the impact of cancer
- fear that the cancer hasn't actually gone and confusion as to how the medical team can know, with certainty, that you no longer have any cancer in you
- sadness at what you've been through, what you've lost and how you've changed
- guilt that you've reached the end of treatment whilst other people (some whom you may know and others you don't know) have either died from cancer or have incurable cancer
- disappointment that despite being told that treatment has been successful, there's no guarantee that the cancer won't come back

- helplessness and a lack of control: if you couldn't control the growth of the cancer within your body in the first place, how can you control it from coming back?
- a feeling of living on borrowed time together with a passionate need to live life to its fullest and best
- anxious feelings, thoughts and emotions which extend beyond cancer and into normal day-to-day life
- loss and grief about the things you've lost during cancer treatment, whether this is the loss of the ability to have children, the loss of a chunk of your life or the loss of friendships
- fear that the cancer will come back, and that it will come back as incurable cancer
- a need to return to normal life but an uncertainty as to what is normal life
- anger at getting cancer; anger at what you've had to go through; and anger at the impact it's had on your life
- a loss of confidence in yourself and a loss of trust in your body
- a feeling that you are a stranger in your own body
- self-loathing and disgust at changes to your physical appearance
- frustration at trying to build yourself back together after treatment only to keep coming across hurdles and difficulties in the process
- overwhelmed and confused: your brain might be overwhelmed with spiralling, uncontrollable thoughts
- guilt for putting your family through the stress of your cancer; guilt at not being able to be 'you' as you went through treatment; guilt at getting cancer in the first place; and guilt for being a burden to friends
- flashbacks to particularly stressful times during treatment and at the point of diagnosis
- a feeling of depletion and generally feeling drained from all the difficult emotions and feelings
- disorientation and feeling like you no longer fit in where you used to feel comfortable – be that with friends or at work
- that you are having an internal struggle between who you were before cancer, who you are now and who you want to be
- uncertainty about how to move forward with your life.

There are so many emotions and feelings swimming around at this stage. Sometimes these emotions and feelings are all jumbled together in one big squishy mush and it can be hard to pinpoint exactly what's going on. You may not be used to experiencing these sorts of emotions and feelings, and a lot of them might be completely new to you. You may not be able to label how you're feeling, why you're feeling a particular way and thus what to do about it. But don't worry, this is all completely normal and perfectly understandable.

Physiological feelings

Accompanying the various emotions, you might also be experiencing some of these physiological – physical – feelings:

- Your stomach might be doing somersaults.
- You may have butterflies constantly in your tummy.
- You may be going to the toilet more often or feeling nauseous.
- Your heart might be thumping in your chest so loudly that you think other people might hear it.
- Your breathing might be shallow or you might keep catching your breath.
- You could be feeling tingly or shaky.
- You might be getting headaches and a tightness in your chest.
- You might find yourself crying for no reason, crying uncontrollably and crying for days on end.

Lingering physical side-effects

And on top of any physiological feelings, you may still have some lingering uncomfortable or painful physical side-effects from treatment, like:

- intense fatigue
- debilitating brain fog
- pain or discomfort from surgery
- radiotherapy reactions to the skin
- bone and joint pain from chemotherapy or hormone therapy
- hot flushes from hormone therapy or an induced menopause
- lymphoedema
- cording from auxiliary node clearance
- peripheral neuropathy
- scar pain or discomfort.

Coping

That's a hell of a lot to have to cope with. And it's a hell of a lot to have to cope with all at the same time. And it's a hell of a lot to have to cope with after your body has very recently been through the cancer-mill! I mean, even if you're just experiencing a few things from each of those three lists, it's a huge amount to deal with.

Dealing with the physical, emotional and mental impact of having had cancer takes time and energy – but there isn't always much of this after treatment. Yes okay, I know you're no longer going to hospital as frequently, but that just means that regular life and regular responsibilities are starting up again: back to work; back to walking the dog; back to the school run; back to food shopping; back to preparing meals; back to everything that either you had help with or didn't get done whilst you went through treatment. How can you possibly process the emotional fall-out of treatment and the lingering physical side-effects while you're trying to grapple with everything that regular life brings with it?

And what about everything else that forms part of regular life – exercising, returning to your personal interests and seeing family and friends? You're probably wondering how and when you're ever going to feel up to socializing again – will you ever have the energy to socialize again, and if you do will there still be invitations seeing as you might be turning down more invitations than accepting at the moment?

You might also be feeling slightly awash with cancer. After all, it's been a huge part of your life for the past few months or years while your life has been prescribed by the treatment and the side-effects from treatment. Not only have you talked about and thought about cancer for close to 24 hours a day, it's highly likely that this has been the main topic of conversation with those around you. So, it's unsurprising if you're now feeling defined by cancer.

And whilst all of this is going on, despite feeling far from normal, you're probably trying your best to look normal to those around you. It's likely that you're putting on a positive front – your brave face – for the rest of the world to see, while inside you feel like you're falling apart.

So where on earth do you start, in terms of recovery? Some of the things that you might like to do at this stage are:

- pretend it never happened
- run away
- get drunk
- hibernate
- move to a deserted island
- hide under the bed covers for the foreseeable future
- bury your head in the sand
- escape to the top of a mountain
- eat a lot of cake.

But none of these are a good idea. Cross them all off your to-do list and instead, take a deep breath and ready yourself for the post-treatment stage of recovery. This is a time for you to recover from the physical side-effects of cancer treatment and also the emotional impact of what you've been through.

Recovery

Recovery is about:

- Recognizing what you're struggling with.
- Understanding that it's perfectly natural to struggle in this way.
- Implementing some strategies and tools to help you cope.
- Being kind to yourself and showing yourself compassion.
- Readjusting your expectations and reassessing your priorities.
- Being patient with yourself.
- Seeking professional help when you need it, and not being scared to do this.
- Making sure that cancer is just part of you and doesn't define you.

It takes time and effort to heal physically and emotionally, so be prepared for your recovery to be a gradual process and to involve some work on your part. Don't expect to see a transformation immediately. Lower your expectations of yourself and be kind to yourself. Over time, what might feel completely overwhelming now will gradually feel more manageable and you'll find that you are able to pick up the pieces and put your life back together. Have you heard of the Japanese art of Kintsugi? This is the art of putting broken pottery pieces back together with gold and in doing so, embracing the flaws and imperfections caused by the breakage and creating an even more beautiful piece of art. Keep this in mind as you move through your recovery.

No doubt you'll have lots and lots of questions crowding your brain at the moment, including questions such as:

- How will my life look as I go through this recovery process and beyond?
- Will life go back to the way it was before cancer?
- Will I go back to the person I was before I had cancer?

Well, life after finishing cancer treatment is different for everyone. Think of life after cancer as a scale – similar to the scale I mentioned in the introduction. At one end of the scale there are those people who go back to living their life exactly as it was pre-cancer. They just slot back into their pre-cancer life, almost as if nothing has happened (yep, these people do exist but I assure you that they are in the minority).

At the other end of the scale, you have those who find that there is absolutely no 'back to normal' and instead they find a completely new way of living their life: they want to use this time for change: they may find a new purpose; they may find growth opportunities; they may find enlightenment (again, a minority of people fall within this group).

And then, in between these two ends of the scale is everyone else – it's where most of you sit. You'll fall back into some of the old ways of life whilst recognizing that life isn't quite the same and that some aspects of life are, and will continue to be, different post-cancer. For example, I would place myself firmly in the mid-point of this scale: I still feel like myself in a number of ways but I now have more appreciation for the little things like waking up to a new day every day; I make an effort to slow down and to stop rushing through life as I used to do pre-cancer; and I prioritize being honest with myself, focusing on things within my control and focusing on the present.

There is no right or wrong way to move forward after cancer, it's all up to you. Regardless of how the future looks for you, remember that you are still you. Yes, you might want to use this time to change yourself and your life, but equally you don't need to find growth opportunities, find a new purpose or anything like that. It's absolutely fine to just focus on you and focus on getting yourself back to you.

It's also worth remembering that life is fluid and nothing stays the same forever. You will inevitably change over time and challenges will always appear, but if you have your own personal toolkit of coping strategies, it will help you to cope with anything that life throws at you. Someone once told me about the Buddhist doctrine of 'anicca': this is the idea that the world is in constant flux and that nothing stays the same. Everything is impermanent. It's something that I remind myself of every day.

And, importantly, at every step of the way along your recovery, you'll learn that you are most certainly not alone in how you're feeling. I recall feeling completely shaken at the end of my treatment. Reaching the end of treatment and trying to move on was far more complex than I'd previously imagined and, in many ways, I felt more at sea than I had done during my treatment. Cathy and Nina both experienced similar feelings:

'When I finished treatment for breast cancer, everything was a challenge. Getting up every day was a challenge'.

Cathy

'I felt so elated when I reached the end of my cancer treatment. I went on an amazing holiday to celebrate and after my holiday I went straight back to work. Then everything I'd been through hit me. I started to feel empty, nothing brought me joy and nothing made sense to me. I started questioning my career, whether I was on the same path as some of my friends. I was at rock bottom'.

Nina

So, if you're ready to start the recovery process, join me, a range of experts including an oncologist, a clinical psychologist and a number of counsellors, together with a host of people who've been through – or are still going through – what you're going through, as we help you to navigate life after breast cancer.

2

Finishing treatment and post-cancer follow-up

The process of finishing treatment and how you will be monitored going forward

'When I was coming to the end of my treatment, one of my main concerns was how I was going to be monitored going forwards'.

Taken from Ticking Off Breast Cancer

Whilst this book is about the physical, emotional and mental challenges that you might face after your cancer treatment has ended and you're moving forward with your life, for some of you it can actually be a challenge to understand what final hospital appointments, follow-up appointments and future monitoring that you will have. So, let's start by looking at some of the practicalities of finishing active treatment for breast cancer.

During treatment, focus is often – rightly – on getting through the treatment and not much detailed thought is given to how you'll be discharged from treatment when it all comes to an end and what will happen then. But then as you get closer to the end of your treatment plan, you might start to wonder what will happen after you have the final chemotherapy infusion or the last radiotherapy session. You might begin to think about things such as:

- Will I see the oncologist?
- Will I have a scan?
- Will I be given a date for a follow up appointment in a few months' time?
- Will I still be able to call the breast care nurse or oncology department with concerns?
- What sort of post-treatment support will I be given?

These are all perfectly natural questions, and in fact it's really good to have them. If you know how you'll be monitored after treatment; who to contact and how; what follow-up appointments you'll have; and from where you will get post-treatment support, this will all go some way to providing you with important reassurance as you navigate your way beyond your cancer treatment.

This chapter looks at all of these things. There's quite a lot to consider, so we're going to look at this in four parts, with the insight and assistance of two super knowledgeable women: Lyndel Moore, who is the Deputy Divisional Director-Head of Cancer Services Integrated and Community Care at the Great Western Hospital Foundation Trust; and Dr Sophie McGrath who is a Consultant Breast Cancer Oncologist at the Royal Marsden NHS Foundation Trust Hospital. We're going to look at the following four common questions in turn:

- How will I be signed off from treatment?
- Did the treatment work?
- How will I be monitored for signs of further cancer?
- What sort of post-treatment support will I receive from now on?

How will I be signed off from treatment?

Okay, so let's start with one of the most important questions that you might have as you near the end of treatment: how will you be signed off from treatment once the active treatment is over? You've been having treatment for what feels like forever: you've had your surgery and completed your course of radiotherapy, biotherapy, immunotherapy and/or chemotherapy and whilst some of you might be continuing with ongoing medication at home like hormone therapy, you no longer have to go to hospital to have treatment. So, you might well be wondering how you will transition away from the hospital, where you've spent a large proportion of your recent weeks and months.

There isn't a straightforward answer to this question because the answer depends on the way things are done at your hospital: hospitals differ in the way they approach the end of treatment transition whereby you are checked over before you're sent on your way, no longer as a cancer patient. Some of you may be given an appointment with your oncologist who will check you over, look at your blood counts and other data, check how any ongoing treatment is going – such as hormone therapy – explain the monitoring and follow-up procedure and provide information about post-treatment support. Some of you may be given an appointment with the clinical nurse specialist for oncology – the breast clinical nurse specialist, a senior oncology nurse or the breast care nurse – at which you'll be given some information about monitoring, follow-up and post-treatment support. Some of you may be at hospitals where you'll see both the oncologist and nurse who will each cover different aspects of this information. And in some circumstances, hospitals may not offer either of these types of appointments at the end of treatment. In that case it is certainly worth requesting an appointment with either the oncologist or appropriate oncology nurse – you never know, they might give you an appointment even though they're not offered as routine.

You might be interested to know that in the UK there is some guidance[1] on the way that breast cancer patients should be monitored and followed up, including the sorts of appointments and information that should be offered to them at the end of their active treatment. It won't surprise you to know that some hospitals have implemented the guidance whilst others haven't. And of those hospitals which have implemented the guidance, they have done so in different ways. So, it's always worth asking your medical team, as you near the end of treatment, what will happen for you once you complete your treatment.

It's important to note that it's quite possible that how you finish treatment and move forward with monitoring and follow-ups might be slightly different to how someone else who has been through their breast cancer treatment at the same hospital finishes treatment and moves forward with monitoring and follow-ups. This is because everyone's breast cancer diagnosis, treatment, and general situation is different. For example, a 20-year-old woman with invasive triple negative breast cancer may well have a different follow-up experience to a 60-year-old woman with non-invasive oestrogen positive breast cancer.

If you have an appointment with your oncologist and/or oncology nurse at the end of your treatment, it's worth going to this appointment with a list of questions about monitoring and follow-ups to make sure that you remember to ask everything. I've put a list of questions into the checklist at the end of this chapter that you could use as a starting point.

Did the treatment work?

As part of your transition away from the hospital at the end of your treatment, it's highly likely that you'll have some questions about the efficacy of your treatment. I mean, the whole point of cancer treatment is to get rid of the cancer and you'll want to know that it's been 100 per cent successful, won't you? It would be totally normal for you to be wondering about things along the lines of:

- How do the doctors know that the treatment has been successful and that it's safe to complete my cancer treatment?
- Will I be given a scan or a test to check that the treatment has been successful: that they've got all the cancer out of me and can't see anything left?
- Is there a blood test or scan that I can have to confirm that there are no stray cancer cells floating about inside me?
- Is there a guarantee that the cancer isn't going to come back?
- What terminology will they use? Will they say 'all clear', 'in remission' or 'cured'?

If you have a final oncology appointment, then the chances are that the oncologist will talk to you about these issues as a matter of course. But for those of you who are not given a final oncology appointment, these questions and their answers are discussed below. Of course, they're covered in a generalized way below, and are not specific to individual situations so it's important to address any personal questions or concerns with your medical team.

So, taking each of the four questions in turn, first up is:

How do the doctors know that the treatment has been successful and that it's safe to complete my cancer treatment?

It's perfectly natural to question how the doctors can be sure that the treatment was successful: that they removed all the cancer and know that there are no stray cancer cells still floating around your body. This is probably the question at the forefront of everyone's mind as they near the end of their cancer treatment – it was certainly at the top of my list of questions. After all, isn't this what all the horrific treatment has been about? Take Fi and Gabi for example. Having very recently completed her breast cancer treatment, Fi told me:

> 'I finished my treatment two weeks ago and I am so worried that the treatment hasn't caught all the cancer. How does my oncologist know that the treatment was a success? I've got a mammogram and follow-up appointment in a week and a half and I'm convinced that they'll find more cancer in my breast. I can't bear the thought of going through everything again'.

And Gabi said about this stage:

> 'When I finished treatment, I wondered how my oncologist knew that the treatment had worked because I didn't have a scan to check. I had aches and pains everywhere so I was convinced that all the cancer hadn't been caught'.

What usually happens (and this can vary depending upon the type, grade and stage of cancer) is that once you've had the cancer taken out of you and some possible mopping up treatment (to catch any stray cancer cells that may have spread beyond your lymph nodes) oncologists can generally state with a fairly high level of certainty (because of medical research, clinical trials and experience) that if you've been given the appropriate treatment for the type of cancer you have, it's highly likely that the treatment will have worked to remove the cancer and to mop up any stray cancer cells.

Some of you might not be entirely clear what your cancer treatment was doing – for example was your chemotherapy mopping up stray cancer cells or was it specifically targeted at your tumour? You were probably told this at the start of your treatment plan, but it was quite possibly at a point when you were in shock and you may not have taken it all in. So, it might be helpful to have a bit of a recap at this stage. You could ask your oncologist for an explanation of what each of the treatments has done: which treatment targeted the tumour, which treatment mopped up stray cancer cells and which treatment has helped minimize the risk of the cancer returning. Knowing this will help give you reassurance that the treatment you were given has helped get rid of the cancer and minimize the risk of it returning.

The second question that you might have is:

Will I be given a scan or a test to check that the treatment has been successful: that they've got all the cancer out of me and can't see anything left?

Whilst you might think that it would help to put your mind at rest to have a scan at the end of treatment – to check that the treatment was successful and to confirm that there is no evidence of disease – it turns out that it's not usual practice in the UK for someone who's had breast cancer to be given a scan as a matter of course. Yes, I know that this can come as a bit of a disappointment for many of you – it was certainly a disappointment for me. But given the impact on the body from a scan – such as radiation – scans are generally not given at the end of treatment unless the patient is showing any symptoms requiring investigation.

For some of you, this may lead to uncertainty or fear that not all the cancer has gone. But it's worth going back to the answer to the previous question. Remember, that given the extensive clinical research and evidence-based treatments given to breast cancer patients, oncologists know, with a high level of certainty, that your type of breast cancer can be successfully treated by the treatment that you've been given. So, if you're showing no symptoms requiring further investigation at this stage, then your oncologist will generally deem that there is no call for a scan.

It's worth noting that, even though it is not usual practice to have a scan as you complete treatment, you'll probably be given a physical examination by your oncologist or breast surgeon at the end of treatment. This is to check your chest area/breasts/reconstructed breasts/under your arms/ lymph nodes for irregular lumps, tissue thickening and skin tethering – especially new changes – that may suggest a recurrence of the cancer (recurrence is covered in more detail in Chapter 5).

The third common question is:

Is there a blood test or scan that I can have to confirm that there are no stray cancer cells floating about inside me?

Oh, wouldn't it be comforting if there was a test to check that there were no stray cancer cells floating around your body that could lead to a spread or recurrence of cancer? But, unfortunately, as at the time of writing this book, in most situations there is no conclusive test to check that there are no stray cancer cells floating around. The assertion that all the cancer has been mopped up and there are no stray cells floating around is based on the knowledge that the treatment you've been given is known to get rid of your type of cancer and minimize the chance of it coming back.

The fourth question that you might ask at this stage is:

Is there a guarantee that the cancer isn't going to come back?

This was a big issue for me, and I recall being distraught at the thought that after having been through all the treatment, there was no 100 per cent guarantee that cancer would not come back. Unfortunately, this is just a fact of life. However, the treatment that you've been given will include whatever treatment is available to help minimize the risk of it coming back. Given that there is no certainty that the cancer will not come back, it's important to be educated about the signs and symptoms to look out for and how to contact the hospital if you're concerned about something. This is covered in more detail below within the section: How will I be monitored for signs for further cancer?

It's worth mentioning here, the NHS online tool called Predict.[2] You may have heard about this tool in your discussions with your oncologist, or even with other women who've had breast cancer. This is a tool that is used by oncologists in their discussions with patients about how breast cancer treatments after surgery might improve the survival rate of the patient. Essentially, the tool predicts the patient's five-, ten- and fifteen-year survival rates on the basis of their current treatment and then their five-, ten- and fifteen-year survival rates with any specific additional treatment. So, for example, it might show that a patient has a 90 per cent chance of surviving ten years on the basis of the treatment they have had to date, but if given Tamoxifen, they would have, say, a 95 per cent chance of surviving for ten years. There would then be a discussion between patient and oncologist about the benefits of taking Tamoxifen versus not taking it. Equally, the tool might calculate that the benefit of a patient having chemotherapy is merely a 3 per cent increase in survival rate for ten years which might suggest to the oncologist that the risks and side-effects of chemotherapy outweigh the benefits of chemotherapy.

Whilst it's a helpful tool for oncologists to use in ascertaining the benefits of certain treatments, the ancillary by-product of this tool is that it can give a patient an indication of their chances of surviving five, ten- and fifteen-years post-treatment. But before you head off to ask your oncologist to use this tool to tell you the statistical chance that you'll survive the next 15 years, here are a few very important words of caution:

- The survival predictions in this tool are based on data from similar women in the past. According to the Predict website, Predict was originally developed using data from over 5000 women with breast cancer. Its predictions were then tested on data from another 23,000 women from around the world to make sure that they gave as good an estimate as possible.
- The tool does not take into account personal factors such as fitness levels, other health issues and lifestyle factors, all of which impact life expectancy. It is a one-size-fits-all tool, but in reality, every breast cancer patient is individual with an individual biology.
- The tool works by entering certain details of a patient's cancer such as the type of cancer, age, menopausal status, oestrogen receptor status, HER2 status, progesterone receptor status, tumour grade and size and lymph node involvement. However, it cannot be used for instances of more than one tumour or no tumour (such as occult breast cancer). It also doesn't take into account the extent of the oestrogen involvement, but rather only whether the cancer is oestrogen positive or negative. Likewise, with lymph node involvement it doesn't take account the size of the lymph nodes, but only the number of nodes involved. All of these factors will have an impact on the chances of surviving for certain lengths of time.
- It provides a guide and not a guarantee.

I can't emphasize enough that it is of paramount importance that you think long and hard about whether you want to know these statistics – once you've heard your statistics, you can't un-hear them.

And last – but by no means least – is the question:

What is the appropriate terminology to use at this stage? Am I 'all clear', 'in remission' or 'cured'?

This is confusing, isn't it? I expect you've heard people using all these terms and you're wondering why some people are told one thing whilst you've been told another. Well, there is no standard terminology that all oncologists use at the end of treatment for primary breast cancer and terminology is often used interchangeably. At the point in time when treatment comes to an end, you will most likely be told that there is 'no evidence of disease' in your body, or 'NED' for short. However, you might find that you are told by your oncologist that you are 'in remission' or 'all-clear'. Part of the confusion is that some oncologists and surgeons use the word 'cured' whilst others don't use this word (favouring instead, the use of terms such as NED). Why some medics used 'cured' whilst others don't, is beyond the remit of this book, but it's worth pointing out here that for the most part, these terms (NED, 'in remission', 'all-clear' and 'cured') are generally interchangeable and if you're confused by the terminology that your consultant has used, it's important to ask him/her to explain it to you.

How will I be monitored for signs of further cancer?

Given that there is no 100 per cent guarantee that the cancer will not come back (although remember that the treatment you've had will all help minimize this risk), it's likely that you'll want to know how you will be monitored going forward for signs of cancer coming back. Again this depends on your hospital procedure.

There are, generally speaking, two ways in which breast cancer patients may be monitored and followed-up after their treatment in the UK. In some hospitals breast cancer patients are given routine follow-up appointments at specific times after their treatment, for example, at six months, one year, two years and so on. These appointments may be a mix of oncology appointments and routine scans (such as mammograms). This is the more traditional method of follow-up.

On the other hand, some hospitals have a patient-initiated follow-up process (often called 'Open Access Follow-Up'). This type of follow-up procedure has been implemented in accordance with the UK guidance that I mentioned earlier in this chapter. Hospitals with a patient-led follow-up process do not give patients routine follow-up appointments at specific times following treatment but rather the onus is on patients to monitor themselves and get in touch with the hospital if they notice anything of concern. Hospitals that have this type of follow-up process will have procedures in place for the patient to easily get in touch with the hospital if they have any concerns and then to get an appointment in the breast clinic at the hospital within a short time frame. It's usual for hospitals following such a process to still provide regular routine mammograms for a certain period of time following treatment.

The patient-led follow-up process might initially sound a little bit more unsettling than having specifically timed post-treatment appointments – after all, knowing that you'll be seeing an oncologist at regular intervals over the next few years may be comforting to some – but research and evidence carried out in the UK[3] has shown that patient-led follow-up is a better method. According to the research, as the onus is on the patient to monitor themselves for signs and symptoms of anything concerning, it encourages the patient to be aware of any changes and to get them checked out straight away rather than waiting for the next routine appointment. Waiting to get changes and concerns checked out at a forthcoming routine appointment risks a delay in getting things investigated and dealt with. It's also been shown that not having set follow-up appointments reduces anxiety for the patient as they are not going through the anxiety associated with the lead up to a routine appointment.

If your hospital follows a patient-led follow-up procedure, the key for you is knowing that the onus is on *you* to monitor for any changes, and for *you* to have the confidence to get back in touch with the hospital at any time with any concerns. The aim is that you will move on from treatment with the reassurance that if you notice any changes or symptoms causing concern, you can contact the hospital knowing that you will be given an appointment in the breast clinic within a short period of time.

In reality, many hospitals have a process that combines both of these approaches – some routine appointments, whilst the patient is also expected to contact the hospital with any concerns or health issues.

Given the disparity between how different hospitals monitor and follow-up their breast cancer patients, it's important that you find out how you will be monitored going forward. This will help provide you with the reassurance that if you have any concerns down the line, you know exactly how to get in touch with the hospital. The sorts of questions that you might like to ask your medical team about the monitoring process, are:

- Will I be having any follow-up appointments and if so, when? Are these at certain specific points post-treatment and how do I get the appointments? Does the hospital generate these appointments for me and then send me a letter with the details, or do I need to call the hospital to make the appointments?
- How do I get back in touch with the hospital with any concerns that I may have?
- What's the process for getting an appointment in the hospital breast clinic if I notice any worrying changes?

Regardless of the hospital procedure, it's really important to understand what you're looking for in terms of changes for which you should seek medical advice. Generally speaking, there are three ways in which breast cancer can 'come back'. Breast cancer can come back as a local recurrence (where you have a tumour near the location of the original tumour); a new incidence of breast cancer (where you have a tumour in the other breast/area of the chest or a tumour in a different part of the breast to where you previously had one); or secondary breast cancer (where the cancer has spread to other parts of the body and which is incurable cancer). So, it's important to be aware of the signs and symptoms of a recurrence/new occurrence of primary breast cancer and the signs and symptoms of secondary breast cancer. I'm not going to go into detail about these here, Chapter 5 provides more information about the types of recurrence and what to look out for in relation to each of the three ways it can come back.

What sort of help and support will be given to me to help me cope with life after cancer?

Once treatment has been completed and you've been signed-off from your treatment (subject to any on-going treatment such as hormone therapy), it's quite common to experience a range of challenging emotions and feelings about what you've been through, how you're presently feeling and generally moving forward with your life. You've just been through a traumatic life experience so it's natural that there will be an impact. After all, it's why you're reading this book. But in addition to understanding what you're going through and how to deal with it, it's perfectly natural to be wondering what sort of local or online support is available to help you during this stage of your recovery.

As with everything else, this all depends on your hospital. Some hospitals have a good range of post-cancer support services whilst other hospitals don't have anything. Some hospitals provide information about post-cancer support services that are available through other channels – such as local charities – whilst other hospitals do not offer such information. It's all very – frustratingly – inconsistent. If you're not given much – or any – information about the availability of post-treatment support, don't worry. There's plenty of post-treatment support out there but you're going to have to find it yourself. This may sound daunting but really, it's not. It's a question of knowing where to look and here are some tips:

- Think about what sort of post-treatment support you need, as you need it. Your needs will change over time so what you might require now, could be different to the support you need in say six months' time.
- If you have access to the breast care nurse or oncologist at your hospital, ask them for information about the support services available at the hospital – if any – and locally. What local support services are available? Do they have a leaflet listing the details of local services?
- Talk to your doctor. Doctors and family physicians often know about the local cancer support services and post-treatment offerings in your local area.
- Talk to any friends you've made during your cancer treatment – are they getting support from anywhere? Can they tell you about any resources in your area?
- Research local charities and cancer support centres – are there any breast cancer support groups or general support groups for people with all types of cancer? What about local cancer or breast cancer charities which provide counselling services?
- Are there any day hospices locally? Don't be put off by the word 'hospice'. Yes, a hospice is often associated with end-of-life care, but in actual fact many day hospices provide support services for people like you who have finished treatment.

21

- Social media can be helpful, if you feel up to looking on it. You'll find lots of people going through exactly the same thing that you're going through. There are also various private Facebook support groups and you'll find that plenty of charities and support services publish social media posts with helpful advice and support.
- Post-treatment support can take many different forms but the sorts of things you might like to look for are:
  - one-to-one counselling sessions
  - group therapy sessions
  - moving forward courses, for example the Maggie's 'Where Now?' course and the Breast Cancer Now 'Moving forward' course
  - relaxation offerings, such as reiki, reflexology, mindfulness and breathing techniques
  - local post-cancer groups for rambling, walking, rowing, dragon boating or fly-fishing
  - post-cancer exercise support such as gyms, personal trainers and fitness centres – these often offer post-cancer classes and sessions whilst some gyms provide a series of free sessions for people who've had cancer
  - exercise sessions provided by national charities – they sometimes put on yoga, Pilates and other exercise/strengthening classes online via their websites so you can do these classes in your own home, or in person at one of their centres if you happen to live near one of their centres
  - post-cancer courses in writing, drawing, painting and other forms of expressive art
  - post-cancer talks on a range of healthy lifestyle topics such as nutrition and exercise
  - support for the physical impact of cancer such as pain management, scar tissue massage, physiotherapy, acupuncture, manual lymphatic drainage for lymphoedema and monitoring your bone health.

Information on the availability of such support can often be obtained from your hospital, your doctor, any local cancer charities/centres, local day hospices, social media, and national charities. The Useful Resources section at the back of the book provides details of some of the particularly helpful national charities that are worth looking at.

Top tip

Make sure you know how to get back in touch with the breast cancer team at your hospital with any concerns you have going forward, and don't be afraid to call them with any concerns you may have.

Checklist

This is a checklist of questions that you might want to ask your oncologist at your final appointment.

As a general note it's worth pointing out that oncologists don't treat all patients the same in terms of how they talk to patients, what they say and the level of detail they go into. There is an element of judgement which goes into how oncologists talk to patients. For example, if a patient is showing signs of wanting a lot of information, then the oncologist might be more forthcoming, but if a patient appears overwhelmed and stressed, the oncologist might not give as much information – choosing to provide only the absolutely necessary information so as to not increase the patient's stress. So, it's vitally important to actually ask the questions you want the answers to.

1 When will I next have a scan? Will it be a mammogram or another type of scan?
2 How often will I have routine scans?
3 How do I get an appointment for my routine scans: do I make an appointment or is an appointment made for me by the hospital?
4 What is the follow-up procedure that the hospital follows for breast cancer patients?
5 Is there a patient-led follow-up process? Or routine oncology appointments?
6 Will I be having any follow-up oncology appointments and if so, when? Are these at certain specific points post-treatment and how do I get the appointments? Are they made for me and I am notified or do I need to call the hospital to make the appointments?
7 Will I still be able to call the breast care nurse or oncology department with concerns?

8　How do I get back in touch with the hospital with any concerns that I may have? Ask for contact details and make sure you know the process for getting an appointment if you have any concerns.

9　What's the process for getting an appointment if I notice any concerning changes?

10　What are the signs and symptoms that I need to keep a lookout for, including secondary breast cancer?

11　What sort of post-treatment support is available from the hospital?

12　What post-cancer support is available locally, outside the hospital, including details of local and national cancer and breast cancer support that the hospital is able to recommend.

Notes

Use this page to make notes of the questions that you have for your medical team about your post-treatment support

3

The loss of a safety net and lack of purpose

Losing the safety net of being in constant contact with the hospital and experiencing a lack of purpose at the point when treatment comes to an end

'Ending treatment and not having to go to hospital is a double-edged sword. It's nice not to have to keep going to hospital but I felt abandoned by the hospital once I stopped my regular visits. When I was in active treatment, I was in regular contact with doctors and nurses and I was always well-informed as to what I was doing in terms of my treatment. But now, post-treatment, I feel like I'm in a no-man's land of not knowing who I should speak to about certain things'.

Molly

So now we're going to move onto the post-treatment challenges that someone may experience when they finish their cancer treatment, and I guess a good place to start is with two challenges that can – for many people – present themselves straight away. That is firstly, losing what feels like a safety net of contact with the hospital; and secondly feeling like you've lost your purpose.

Loss of the hospital safety net

It's actually very common to feel that you've just lost your safety net when you no longer need to regularly go to hospital for treatment. After all, going to hospital on a regular basis where you're looked after and listened to, can feel like a wonderfully supportive safety net ready to catch you at any moment. In fact, the hospital, and everything that it provides, can feel like a life raft in the choppy sea of cancer. Oncologists, surgeons, radiographers and nurses are all looking after you and looking out for you during what is, arguably, one of the most vulnerable periods of your life.

The medics are actively doing something to your body to get rid of the cancer, whether that is cutting it out, administering radiation or pumping chemotherapy drugs into your bloodstream. And on top of this, they're regularly checking your physical state with their tests and examinations: blood tests and scans are undertaken to see what is going on inside you, checking that the bad cells have gone and have not reappeared or spread.

Not only are all these wonderful medics monitoring your physical welfare, they, and their colleagues, are also keeping an eye on your emotional well-being and mental state by talking to you, checking you're feeling okay and listening to your worries and fears. Someone is usually there (in person or on the phone) to talk to about any concerns you have, whether it's a question about how to manage the side-effects, a concern about your treatment plan, or just getting some reassurance about everything you're going through. And there's always an upcoming appointment at which you can raise any worries or ask any questions.

But then, treatment ends and you no longer need to visit the hospital on such a regular basis, if at all. The cancer has been taken out and depending upon the grade, stage and spread of your cancer, you may have had some treatment to mop up any stray cancer cells and you might now be on some form of medication which aims to reduce the risk of the cancer returning. You've probably been told something along the lines of there being no evidence of disease in you;[1] that you'll be due to return to hospital for a check-up in, say, six or twelve months;[2] and that you're now free to go. Having been enclosed in the warm embrace of the cancer ward, you're now on your own, and it can certainly feel like you've been cast adrift.

Being cast adrift from the hospital can feel distressing and, quite honestly, terrifying. It can be pretty scary when you're no longer going for regular appointments and no longer in regular contact with the nurses and doctors. If this all strikes a chord with you, and you're struggling with letting go of the hospital safety net, you are most certainly not alone. Many people feel this way: take Gabi and Jo H for example.

'While I was going through treatment, I was desperate not to be a patient. But when I finished treatment and was no longer a patient I was desperately trying to cling onto the doctors and nurses for reassurance. I was in contact with the hospital every few days: I had an amazing support network around me. If I had any questions about what I was going through, there was always someone to ask. But now, I feel like I am standing at the edge of the cliff without a safety net'.

Gabi

'When I finished treatment, I felt very alone. One minute you are backwards and forwards to the hospital and the next minute you are left to your own devices. I found this time the most difficult'.

Jo H

So, what can you do to help yourself at this point? Well, let's look at some strategies for coping with the loss of the hospital safety net, with some very helpful insight and advice from Barbara Babcock who is a Coach and Trainee Family Therapist. Barbara has helped coach numerous people navigating post-treatment life and she's got stacks of good advice.

To start with, Barbara says that safety nets are essentially ways of receiving reassurance to make you feel safe, calm and protected. If you feel like you've just lost your safety net, and it's making you feel unsettled, nervous or apprehensive, then she suggests that the best thing that you can do now is to create your own, new safety net. You may be wondering how you might do that. Well, she says that the key to creating your own safety net is to work out how *you* can reassure yourself at this point in time. It's important to learn how to reassure yourself rather than relying on external sources providing you with reassurance: if you're waiting for other people to reassure you, you risk waiting a long time and then not even getting the reassurance that works for you (and I think we can all relate to that can't we)?

It turns out that most of us actually have a mechanism for reassuring ourselves. The chances are that you might not even know that you're doing it. So, make a cuppa, grab a pen and notebook (or use the notes page at the end of this chapter) and using these suggested prompts from Barbara, take a few moments to think about how, over the course of your life, you generally reassure yourself:

- Has there been a difficult time in your life (other than cancer) where you've had to reassure yourself? How did you do it at that time?
- What sorts of things do you tell yourself when you're facing a challenge?
- What reassuring sentences do you use? Do you say things like 'We've got this' or 'I've got this'? Interestingly, Barbara says that it's common to tell yourself things like 'We can do this' and 'We've got this' when you're facing a challenge. By using the word 'we' it can help to bring together all your internal resources that can help get through a difficult time – things like your resilience, tenacity and ability to break down a problem into smaller manageable problems.

According to Barbara, you can take those coping mechanisms and the ways that you've reassured yourself in the past, and build them into a whole new safety net that you can take forward with you as you move on from cancer treatment. Brilliant! She also suggests some other things that you can build into this new safety net. Think about the answers to these questions:

- What are your strengths? Consider things like problem solving, being adaptable and having determination.
- What else do you have in your life that makes you feel safe? This might include a supportive partner, a roof over your head, food on the table or a job providing an income.
- Which everyday routines make you feel reassured? Think about things like doing the school run and knowing that the children have been dropped off at school safely; going for a run and knowing that your body is capable of exercising; or making a meal knowing that you have enough food for the family.
- Who is in your support network of friends and family on whom you can call in times of need to ask for help? Do you have a particular friend or group of friends who you can talk to about anything that might be worrying you?

Why not use the notes page at the end of this chapter (or your notebook) to consider these questions and how you can build these things into your new safety net.

One of the trickiest aspects of losing your safety net, is suddenly not having easy access to the hospital and your medical team to ask any number of questions – you know, those middle-of-the-night questions that keep going around your head that you can ask your oncologist at the next appointment; or your chemo nurse at the next infusion; or your breast care nurse at any time because she's given you her on-call number for any and all questions and concerns. What on earth can you do to cope with what feels like having the rug pulled out from under your feet?

Well, Barbara suggests that it's helpful – and important – to ascertain when and where you might get medical advice or assistance now that your treatment has come to an end. Rather than focusing on the fact that you no longer have your usual avenues to access advice and assistance, now is the time to work out where you can go for help and assistance. Some of the things that Barbara suggests you could include in your post-cancer health safety net are:

- Ensure that you know exactly how you will be monitored going forward and what the follow-up procedure is for you. If in doubt, ask your oncologist, breast care nurse or surgeon. Chapter 2 gives some guidance on the ways in which hospitals often monitor and follow-up with patients once their treatment has ended.
- Find out who you can talk to at the hospital about any post-cancer health issues and worries and make sure you keep the telephone number in your phone. Is there a telephone number for an oncology nurse whom you can continue to call with any questions? Ask your medical team about this because you never know, there might be someone. The checklist at the end of Chapter 2 sets out some questions to ask your medical team at the end of treatment and the answers to these will be really helpful in creating your new safety net.
- Research where else you can turn for specific post-cancer advice. Many charities have advice lines and support groups. Record the numbers in your phone, or make a note of them, knowing that you can call them with any post-cancer related issues. The Useful Resources section at the back of the book has a list of national charities that provide this sort of advice, but it's also worth looking for local cancer support groups and centres.
- Always put future appointments in your diary or calendar so that you know when you are next due for a follow up.
- Between follow-up appointments, make a note of any questions that you want to ask at your next appointment. For urgent questions that can't wait until the next appointment, you can call one of the charity advice lines, make an appointment with your physician, doctor, or call the hospital number if you've been given one for these situations.
- Barbara says that it's important to recognize that whilst peer support is invaluable and can give you reassurance, don't rely on your peers (friends, family and social media) for medical information.

Just a little note about *certainty* and *control* here. I dare say that you're craving the return of certainty and control in your life now that you're out of treatment and trying to get your life back to some semblance of the way it was before cancer. You may think that your new safety net should include *certainty*. We all know that certainty can be achieved by control, so therefore you may feel that you need to be more in control of your life. However, just a few words of advice from Barbara on this: she warns that after cancer treatment, there can be a tendency to try to control everything in your life, but this can be unhealthy and lead to more problems so you should just be aware of this and aim to achieve a healthy balance of control in your life.

Lack of purpose

Not only can you feel like you've lost your safety net when you no longer regularly visit the hospital for treatment, but – as I explained back at the start of this chapter – you might also feel that you've lost an important purpose in your life, and this can feel quite destabilizing. Let me explain …

Being told that there is cancer inside you is terrifying. The immediate reaction for most people is usually something along the lines of, 'get it out of me'. And this is the whole point of cancer treatment – to get the cancer out of you and help minimize the risk of it coming back. To totally rely on others to do this, when it's your body, may cause you to feel exposed and vulnerable. So naturally, in order to counter these feelings of exposure and vulnerability, you'll probably take on the treatment with a purpose. Whether this is ticking appointments off a list, reading up on treatment and asking your oncologist questions, keeping yourself healthy between appointments, or just getting yourself to and from every one of those innumerable hospital appointments, you're being proactive. It's a team effort: you and the medical team. You have created a purpose for yourself during treatment: to actively help the medics to rid your body of cancer.

And then the treatment stops. One moment you're having some chemotherapy drugs pumped into your veins or you're having radiation targeted at part of your body, and the next moment you're at home having a cup of coffee with no hospital appointments for the foreseeable future. There are no more appointments to tick off, you've asked all the questions you can ask about the course of treatment, and you no longer have to get yourself to hospital on a regular basis. So, what do you do now? What's your purpose now?

Maybe you feel overwhelmed by this lack of direction and unsure how to adjust to no longer having that purpose in your life. Maybe you feel let down by the hospital – after becoming such a regular visitor and feeling like part of the furniture, you're suddenly left to your own devices. Maybe you have absolutely no idea what to do or how to think without your medical team telling you what to do or what to think. Maybe you're thinking: *What the hell do I do now?*

Well, I can tell you that you're most definitely not the only one feeling this way: it's very common to experience these sorts of feelings. Take Jo H and Mary for example. When I talked to them about this stage of finishing treatment, Jo H told me:

> 'One minute I was on auto-pilot, going backwards and forwards to the hospital without a spare moment to think of anything other than getting through each step of treatment and onto the next. And the next minute I felt that I was left to my own devices and I just wasn't sure how to navigate this stage'.

And Mary explained:

> 'All the time I was going through treatment, I had a big whiteboard in the kitchen. I wrote all the hospital appointments on this whiteboard and I crossed them off as I worked through them. It was my purpose, my direction. I was travelling towards the end of my treatment – it was all I could think about. But then I finished my last radiotherapy session and it felt like a real anti-climax. I just didn't know what to do with myself'.

So what can you do to help with this feeling of uncertainty, lack of purpose/control and general discombobulation? Well, thankfully we have Barbara to help us with this. She says:

> 'Just like now is the time to create a new safety net, now could also be the time to create a new purpose. You had a purpose during treatment and you've fulfilled that purpose. Now it's time for a new phase of your life and with this, a new purpose. But the purpose you give yourself now will not last forever, it will evolve, adapt and change over time because everyone's purpose in life is constantly evolving, adapting and changing throughout their life'.

Okay, so you need to create a new purpose, but how on earth do you do that? Time for another cup of tea and a quiet spot to do some more thinking and note-taking (so grab your pen again).

Barbara suggests that in thinking about the next purpose for yourself, you could think about how you want to live your life, what are your plans and how do you see yourself achieving these plans? Why not take some time to think about, and even write about, the answers to the following questions?

- What do you want out of life?
- What's important to you?
- If you were living a life that you found meaningful and joyful, what would you be doing? Who would be a part of your life? How would you be feeling? What would be different from the life you live now? What would be the same?
- Where do you see yourself making a contribution? Is this at work, at home or elsewhere?

There are no right or wrong answers to these questions, they are just ways to help you look at your life now. You don't even need to come up with the answers immediately, they are questions to think about over time. In fact, your answers to these questions may change over time so it might be worth thinking about them now and again. As Barbara says, the point of these questions is to help you to become aware of your values and what is important to you so that as you move forward and try to find purpose, you can do so authentically, based on your values and beliefs.

Top tip

Some people find it easy to consider the suggested questions in this chapter on their own, some people like to talk to friends and others want to do it with a therapist or a coach. It might also be helpful to take a look at Chapter 17 which covers the concept of the 'new normal' after cancer and provides some insight and advice on adapting to some of the changes you might be experiencing.

Checklist

Here's a recap of the key points for you to take away from this chapter.

1 It's perfectly normal to feel like you've lost a safety net or that you've lost your purpose when you no longer need to go to hospital after treatment.
2 You can create your own safety net of reassurance once treatment has ended by thinking about your own coping mechanisms and strengths.

3 Knowing that you have a support network of friends and family on whom you can call in times of need, can help make you feel reassured.

4 Ensure that you understand the way in which you will be monitored by the hospital going forward, and how the hospital follow-up procedure works.

5 Make sure you know who is responsible for arranging any follow-up appointments at the hospital – is it you, or are appointments automatically created and notified to you?

6 If you are due to have follow-up appointments, ensure you have all your appointments in the diary.

7 Know who to contact in relation to any health concerns, and how to contact them. This might be the breast care nurse or the oncology team at your hospital. Pop the contact number into your phone.

8 Support from charities and local support services can be an invaluable form of reassurance once treatment has finished – research what is available to you locally, and for a list of national charities see the Useful Resources section at the back of the book.

9 Don't try to control everything in your life now, but rather aim to maintain a healthy balance of control and acceptance.

Notes

Use this page for your notes on creating your new safety net and your new purpose

4

Anxiety

What is anxiety and how to cope with it

'I'm anxious, stressed and withdrawn as a result of having had cancer. It feels like I've had a personality transplant: I'm no longer the fun-loving Cathy that everyone loves to be around'.

Cathy

Along with feeling like you've lost your safety net and direction, it's very common to feel all sorts of other emotions and feelings after cancer treatment: both in the short-term during the weeks and months immediately following the end of treatment, and in the long-term over the years that follow. As I mentioned in the introduction, for many people these are all tangled together in one big messy jumble and it can feel impossible to know what's what. Anxiety is often part of this jumble. It's one of the most common emotions that people experience at this point. It can be such a big part of the tangled jumble that if you can identify it, extract it, understand it and deal with it, you'll find it much easier to deal with the remainder of the jumble.

It's worth pointing out that not everyone can pinpoint what they're feeling and recognize it as anxiety. Whilst some of you may know – from experience, from talking to a medical professional or from doing some research – that what you're experiencing is anxiety, others of you may notice some new overwhelming feelings or emotions and not know that they are 'anxiety'. Whether or not you can label what you're experiencing as anxiety, these feelings and emotions can be scary, overwhelming and cause great distress.

Anxiety is a huge topic (and pretty complicated), so we're just going to cover the basics. But a little heads-up here, even just looking at the basics is a lot to take in because to fully understand how to deal with anxiety it's important to understand why you're feeling anxious. And this involves a little bit of science which might be a bit daunting for some of you but do bear with it because it all helps to put your feelings into context. Thankfully we have a super expert to help us. Dr Jane Clark is a Consultant Clinical Psychologist who specializes in treating people who have had cancer. For those of you who've not come across a psychologist before, they are trained mental health professionals who help people learn healthy ways to handle mental health challenges. They can help people living with specific conditions, like depression or anxiety, or those who are going through a tough time in life, like going through cancer. They undergo years of education and training to be able to provide a range of mental health services.[1] To help explain everything as clearly as possible, this chapter is divided into some manageable sections:

- How anxiety might manifest itself in you and the sorts of anxious feelings, thoughts and emotions that people may experience at the end of treatment, as shown by some personal anecdotes.
- What exactly anxiety is, and why it's entirely natural for you to feel anxious after cancer.
- Some practical tips from Jane, for dealing with anxiety at this stage in your recovery.

How might anxiety manifest itself?

So, first things first, let's look at some of the ways that anxiety can manifest. This will help you to recognize whether it's something that you're experiencing in order to work out how to best deal with it. There are, generally speaking, three ways in which you might experience anxiety: firstly, physically; secondly as thoughts; and thirdly as emotions. Of course, some people can experience all three kinds of anxiety, some people can experience a couple and some people just one of these types of anxiety. Remember, everyone is different.

Physiological anxiety

Let's start with physical anxiety which is what the psychologists call 'physiological anxiety'. Interestingly – and this may surprise some of you – anxiety is not just thoughts and emotions going on in your mind, but it can also be something physical such as sweaty palms, a racing heartbeat, breathlessness, a heaviness in the chest area, sickness, tiredness, shaking, headaches, needing to go to the toilet, trembling and feeling jittery, panicky and irritable. It can even manifest as a physical 'whoosh': something so extreme and so strong that it takes the wind out of your sails.

These physical manifestations of anxiety might occur in response to something going on at a specific moment – such as going for a follow-up appointment at the hospital – or they might occur in response to the build-up of events over time, for example, as a result of being over-whelmed by returning to regular day-to-day life or the fear of a cancer recurrence. And it's important to note that it's not just thoughts about cancer that can trigger physical manifestations of anxiety, it can be thoughts about anything going on in day-to-day life at any point in time.

Sound familiar? It certainly does to me. Fairly soon after I'd finished my treatment, I sometimes felt a heaviness on my chest – like a heavy weight sitting on my chest making it difficult for me to breathe. This heavy weight could remain there for a few days or even weeks. Sometimes the weight got heavier and led to breathlessness and palpitations. And if I didn't manage to calm myself down at that point, I went on to expe-rience a full-blown panic attack with light-headedness, shaking, sweat-ing, over-heating, unable to breathe and uncontrollable sobbing. Not pleasant.

Gabi also experienced physiological anxiety. When I talked to her about anxiety, she said:

> 'For me the anxiety developed into a physical manifestation. For a while I'd been convincing myself that the cancer had returned and that I was going to die – I was experiencing a lot of aches and pains due to the hormone treatment I was taking following treatment and I'd convinced myself that these were a sign that the cancer was back. One evening, I was putting my son to bed and my mind was racing with awful thoughts about dying from cancer and leaving my son without a mother. I'd finished putting him to bed and suddenly my legs went from underneath me and I collapsed. I experienced a physical breakdown as a result of my anxiety'.

Thought-based anxiety

Now let's turn to 'thought-based anxiety' which is where the anxiety is predominantly in your thoughts and you have fewer – if any – physical symptoms. Thought-based anxiety is where you experience spiralling, out of control, catastrophic thoughts. These anxious thoughts are not necessarily related to cancer (such as thoughts about cancer returning) but they could be thoughts about anything going on in life. For example, some people experience anxious thoughts about being a good enough parent, doing well at work or feeling paranoid about what people are saying about them behind their back. Anxious thoughts are racing, uncontrollable and often on a 'worst case scenario' basis.

Kathryn described her anxiety to me as:

'Sometimes during the day, my head races with thoughts about having had cancer. My mind gets overactive with these thoughts and then I start worrying about other things, like going back to work and what would happen if I lose my job. My mind is racing. So, I try to distract myself from these thoughts by shutting myself away and watching the tv or reading a book or looking at my phone. But all this does is to add to the racing thoughts in my head and I end up feeling worse. I know I need to put the brakes on my thoughts but I can't do anything. So, I find myself crying a lot and feeling very emotional'.

And Juliet explained her anxiety to me in this way:

'Cancer brought a lot of anxiety to the surface for me and I struggled with anxious thoughts for some time after treatment. There was one occasion, around two years after treatment, where I had a holiday booked but when it came to it, I couldn't go on it. I just felt so incredibly anxious about leaving the house, my grown-up children and going away. That was the point when I realized, I needed to work on my anxiety otherwise it was going to continue to affect my ability to live my life'.

Emotional anxiety

The third way in which you may experience anxiety is as 'emotional anxiety'. This is where anxiety manifests itself as a feeling, such as a feeling that something really bad is going to happen and there is nothing you can do to prevent it. It's a feeling of being on edge, uneasy, agitated. For example, some people may have a fear of leaving the house whilst others who've never previously experienced claustrophobia find themselves feeling claustrophobic in many situations.

Take Rachel L and Sara, for example. Rachel L described her anxiety to me as:

'Since having cancer, I have increased anxiety, I've become very jumpy and I tend to catastrophize a lot – I visualize disasters around every corner. I can't walk down the stairs without clearly visualizing tumbling down and cracking my head open and when I cross the road, I imagine a car hitting me. It's exhausting'.

And Sara told me:

> 'Since having had cancer, I generally feel more on edge and jumpy. I feel really anxious about my children – who are grown up and have left home – and my husband when I know that they are out. I have a horrible feeling that something bad is going to happen to them. It's an intense feeling and it impacts me on a daily basis – I don't feel settled until I know everyone is safely back at their homes'.

Does any of this sound familiar? If so, you are most certainly not alone because according to Jane, it really is very normal to experience anxiety after cancer. If you're like me, then you'd probably like to know why this is.

What is anxiety?

So, onto the second section of this chapter and this is where we look at what exactly anxiety is. Thankfully we have Jane to help explain things and she's going to take us back to basics and explain why we humans experience anxiety and why cancer causes anxiety. In order to do this, it's time for a quick biology lesson from Jane but don't worry this is far more interesting than biology at school because it actually relates to something that you're currently experiencing: it's fascinating stuff.

According to most experts, human brains have evolved over thousands of years from the brain of the more primal species to become the sophisticated mammalian brain that we have nowadays. A simple model is to think of the brain having an older part and a newer part.

The newer part of the brain is called the pre-frontal cortex. The pre-frontal cortex is the part of our brain that has developed as we have evolved into humans from primates. The pre-frontal cortex is responsible for more rational thinking, for example, it's responsible for planning and creativity.

Now let's look at the older, more primal, part of the human brain. It's this older part of the brain which is responsible for survival: it's home to what is known as the 'human threat system'. The primary function of this threat system has always been to protect us from danger and keep us alive. It's the 'flight, fight or freeze' inbuilt system within us that is always switched on and scanning for danger, and which automatically fires up to full alert under certain circumstances, such as when your life is at risk. The easiest way to explain this is to give you an example.

Consider, for example, the caveman stepping out of his cave. If the caveman saw a sabre-toothed tiger, his threat system would have immediately and automatically reacted to this threat by firing up to full alert and sending signals to either run away (flight), fight the tiger (fight) or hide (freeze). It would have been an instant reaction by the caveman's brain, without conscious thought. And once the caveman had successfully dealt with the tiger threat by fleeing, fighting or freezing, the threat system would calm back down to its vigilance mode – that is to say it would remain switched on in the background, scanning for threats.

Fast forward quite a few years and cancer is today's equivalent of the sabre-toothed tiger. You've been told that you have cancer: you have something inside your body that's going to kill you unless the medical team take it out and give you a stack of treatment. Hearing that you have cancer will cause the threat system in the old part of your brain to automatically fire up to full alert and put you in 'flight, fight or freeze' mode.

As Jane points out, it's important to note that this is an automatic and immediate reaction, which bypasses the newer, more rational part of the brain – the pre-frontal cortex – to give that instant reaction. But unlike the days of the sabre-toothed tiger, you can't run away, physically fight or hide from cancer. You can't successfully deal with the threat in one of the prescribed ways and so instead of calming back down to its vigilance mode – as it would have done had you been able to flee, fight or freeze – the threat system keeps on firing on full alert to remind you of the danger.

You might think that you could give yourself a stern talking to and that you could consciously tell the threat system to switch off – after all it's your brain and you're in control. But no, the threat system is there to protect you and it will override every other part of your brain in order to protect you. Feelings like anxiety are a result of our threat system being activated.

As a result of being unable to both stop the threat system from being on full firing alert mode and put it back into vigilance mode, the threat system can go into overdrive. It's the overdrive of the system that causes chronic anxiety. Anxiety is the body's reaction to being in full alert threat mode.

Biology lesson over and as you can see, experiencing anxiety as a result of cancer is absolutely normal. Your brain is just doing its job. Your threat system has been firing off on full alert in response to your life being in danger. But now that the threat system is firing off on full alert, unable to return to vigilance mode, it's causing these uncomfortable thoughts, feelings and emotions that you're experiencing.

You might be wondering why you're experiencing anxiety now that treatment – and the imminent threat of death – is over. After all, you had your diagnosis quite a while back and yet here you are, alive and with no cancer in you, so why all the anxiety now? It's a good question.

According to Jane, it can be to do with the reassurance provided by the hospital during treatment. Whilst going through treatment you have lots of experts looking after you – experts are checking your blood count, they're looking at your scans and they're checking your overall well-being. You're seeing nurses, oncologists, surgeons, radiographers and a host of other medical experts all the time. However, reaching the end of treatment can instil a feeling of loss and a worry about how to look after yourself, especially in relation to knowing what to look out for with regards to the cancer returning. You no longer have the regular reassurance from the hospital. It's this loss of reassurance, together with having to cope on your own, more time to think and more brain space for all sorts of emotions to rise up, that can cause the threat system to go into overdrive: adrenaline is released and you feel anxious and unsettled.

This is quite a lot to take in, so Jane has a helpful way to explain what's going on. She suggests that you think of your threat system as a smoke detector. You have a smoke detector in your house to protect you from the danger of fire. Imagine that the smoke detector develops a fault and, on an occasion when it goes off in response to the presence of smoke in your house, it doesn't switch off again. You've dealt with the smoke so that there is no longer any smoke in your house, but the smoke detector is still making that loud, shrill, beeping noise. Your threat system after cancer is this faulty smoke detector. It went off – rightly so – when it perceived a danger to your life at the time of your cancer diagnosis. You've had treatment to get rid of the cancer and the imminent threat to your life is over, but the smoke detector keeps going off – filling your body with adrenaline and making you feel anxious.

Are you keeping up? It's quite a lot to grasp, isn't it? But now that you know why you're experiencing anxiety, the next step is to work out how to deal with it and this involves – in technical terms – calming down the threat system from full alert to its normal low-level vigilance status. Or, in terms of the smoke detector – turning off that loud shrill beeping noise.

How to deal with anxiety

Okay, let's turn to the ways in which you can calm your anxiety. Jane explains that the ways in which you can calm your anxiety depends on how your anxiety manifests itself. Remember how earlier in the chapter Jane explained that anxiety can be physiological, thought-based or emotional? Well, we're now going look at each of those in turn. If you can't quite identify which type of anxiety you're experiencing, don't worry. The tips for calming all types of anxiety are very similar and you can practise a selection of the suggested strategies.

Calming physiological anxiety

First up, let's look at how you can calm physiological anxiety. Remember, this is the physical manifestation of anxiety like feeling intense fear, your heart racing, breathing faster, feeling sick, needing the toilet and experiencing a seemingly uncontrollable release of emotion such as, sobbing or intense fear or anger.

The first step in calming down this physiological anxiety is to recognize that these feelings are a result of the fact that you've been through a lot and that, as a result, the threat system in your brain is overworking. It can be helpful to go back to Jane's biology lesson and understand that you can't switch off the threat system but instead you'll need to calm the whole system down. Once you recognize that this is what is going on, you can take steps to rebalance the system.

A quick – but very important – reminder here: be kind to yourself. It's really very important to treat yourself with compassion and kindness. Try not to criticize yourself for the way you're feeling as this can make things even worse. A little trick is to imagine that one of your good friends is in your position, and then think about how you would treat that friend. That's how you should treat yourself right now.

Back to calming down your physiological anxiety and at this point, Jane suggests that it might be helpful to think about a seesaw. Yes, one of those seesaws that you'll probably have been on in the park when you were little where a child sits at either end, bouncing up and down. Just as a seesaw can only tip in one direction at a time, it's impossible to feel both anxious and calm at the same time. There's a little bit more biology here, but if you're like me, understanding what's going on in the brain that's causing the anxiety, can really help with understanding how to calm the anxiety.

At one end of the seesaw is your sympathetic nervous system which is firing off all the chemicals (including adrenaline) that are making you feel the way you do when you feel anxious. And at the other end of the seesaw is your parasympathetic nervous system which is the part of the brain that is responsible for the chemicals that make you feel calm. The aim is to balance the seesaw so that it isn't continually tipped towards the sympathetic nervous system.

If you're experiencing any of the physiological anxiety symptoms then you can recognize that your seesaw is tipped towards the sympathetic nervous system. As you can't switch off the sympathetic nervous system, you need to balance the seesaw by tipping it towards the parasympathetic nervous system. You do this by switching on the parasympathetic nervous system which will calm down the sympathetic nervous system. You can switch on your parasympathetic nervous system doing something that you know will calm you down.

So, how can you calm yourself? How can you 'switch on your parasympathetic nervous system'? Jane's advice is that there is no right or wrong way of calming yourself down – it's all about understanding what works for you in order to feel calm, content and at peace. If you don't know what works for you, then you could try some of these suggestions:

- Slow down your breath. Studies indicate that slowing the breathing rate and taking regular slower breaths, with more emphasis on the outbreath calms down the body and switches on the parasympathetic nervous system. Take a look at the Toolkit at the back of the book for some simple breathing exercises.
- Practise mindfulness – the Toolkit at the back of the book explains mindfulness and provides some mindfulness exercises.
- Do a short, guided meditation. There are plenty of phone Apps with guided meditations. Or look on YouTube – search for 'guided meditation' and you will find lots. Try a few until you find one that feels right for you.
- Try some gentle stretching for five minutes.

- Go for a walk in the fresh air.
- Do some mindful movements like Yoga or Pilates.
- Curl up under a soft blanket with a cup of hot chocolate, watching TV or reading a book.
- Do some gardening.
- Sit down with the dog or cat on your lap and stroke them. There's something incredibly calming about doing this.
- Do something creative like painting, drawing or writing.

The key is to do something that tips the seesaw away from the anxious end to the calm end. If you can work out what tips your seesaw towards the calm end, you can then practise that every time you experience any physiological anxiety.

Jane has a little warning here. It's a bad idea to use comfort eating, drugs and alcohol for tipping your seesaw. It might feel like these things help in the short-term but in the longer-term, they cause more problems. They tend to have a re-bound effect on anxiety as they wear off so your anxiety becomes more intense after the initial period of relief provided by these things. There are also lots of social problems that these coping mechanisms can cause, such as creating issues with family and friends.

It's worth just mentioning panic attacks here. According to Jane, a panic attack can occur when your anxiety builds to a point where you experience a number of intense physiological symptoms such as:

- breathing faster and with shallow snatches of breath;
- feeling light headed, dizzy, unsteady or faint;
- feeling shaky or trembling;
- heart palpitations or beating faster;
- uncontrollable crying;
- feeling like your brain and body are out of your control.

According to Jane, it's important to understand that a panic attack cannot harm you even though it feels like it might. During a panic attack, the adrenaline released into your body will reach a peak at which point it's physiologically impossible to produce more adrenaline. You may feel horrendous, but the adrenaline level will plateau and you will come down from that peak: you will not die from a panic attack. This will feel like a challenge but try to not 'escape' from the panic attack. Don't fear the panic as this makes it worse. If you can stay with it and be curious about what's happening, then you might find that the panic doesn't build so much. Jane's tips for dealing with a panic attack:

- Recognize that what you're experiencing is a panic attack and not anything more serious. It is just an extreme physiological brain response, but you are safe.
- Slow your breathing by taking some slow deep breaths, and focusing on the outbreath, keeping this long and slow. Try counting your breaths.
- Ground yourself by focusing on something like a tree in your sightline, your feet on the floor or the horizon if you can see it.
- Don't try to fight it.
- Know that it will pass, you just need to ride it out.

That was a great deal of information to take in, and it only covered physical anxiety! Let's move on, to how to calm the second type of anxiety: anxious thoughts.

Calming thought-based anxiety

Earlier in the chapter Jane explained that thought-based anxiety is where your thoughts are often spiralling, out of control, catastrophic thoughts. Jane's first piece of advice is that if you're experiencing racing, uncomfortable, scary thoughts then rather than trying to fight these thoughts, or trying to push them back down, just recognize that you're having these thoughts and let them move on. If you try to push the thoughts away, they can sometimes come back stronger, so just notice them and see if you can let them go on by.

For example, if your mind is racing with thoughts about the cancer coming back, notice that you're thinking about this, thank your mind for trying to protect you and then see if you can switch your attention to other things that matter to you, see if you can allow the thoughts to be there but place your focus on the day ahead.

Admittedly it's not as easy to do this as it sounds and it takes a bit of practice. Here are some of Jane's suggestions to help the next time you experience anxious thoughts:

- Picture the anxious thoughts being tied up in a little bag that you can let go of and allow to float away.
- Imagine your thoughts written on leaves and let the leaves float down a stream.

- Imagine your thoughts like clouds in the sky – notice all the different thoughts and how they can move through the sky.
- Sometimes it can be helpful to write down a thought in the middle of a piece of paper. Then add, *'I'm having the thought that ...'* before the thought. Notice how that feels different. Thoughts are not facts (even though they can feel very persuasive) and sometimes that slight separation can help.
- Sometimes it can be helpful to notice how your relationship with thoughts changes throughout the day. What seems so definite and important in the middle of the night can seem so different in the middle of the day. It's the same thought but our relationship to it changes. Does that change the power of the thought? Can you notice and say to yourself, *'Thank you mind for giving me that thought at 3 a.m. when it's more difficult for me to cope with it'*.
- Try to change your thoughts from anxious thoughts to non-judgmental thoughts. For example, instead of thinking, *'I feel so anxious, I'm useless at coping'*, try thinking, *'I'm noticing that I am having some anxious thoughts and I thank my brain for trying to protect me'*.

The key here is to recognize that you're having these thoughts but you're letting them move on. It can be difficult to think in these ways – I can say that from experience – but the more you practise thinking in these ways, the easier it becomes and it really can help.

Calming emotional anxiety

Let's look at how to cope with the third type of anxiety: emotional anxiety. This is the anxious feeling – the feeling of being on edge, agitated and that something is about to go wrong. In this situation you can try to make space for the emotion. Here are Jane's suggestions:

- When an anxious feeling is arriving, try not to fight it but allow it to arrive and try to breathe around it. If you try to force the feeling away or push it back in its box, you risk making the emotion more powerful. Instead, try one of the breathing exercises outlined in the Toolkit at the back of the book.
- You can also try breathing around the emotion. To do this, imagine where the physical representation of the emotion is located in your body. Imagine the emotion is a colour. Picture this coloured

representation of the emotion within your body. Imagine the outline of the shape of the emotion and then notice the spaces around the outside of it. Breathe calmly and notice what happens to the spaces around the shape. Stay with the emotion, allow it to pass and to lose its power.

- Think about your anxiety as waves of emotion. What will help you when the waves are bigger and rougher? Know that the storm will pass and the waves will reduce.
- Remember to be kind and compassionate to yourself. It's tough experiencing these waves of emotions. What do you need to have in place to help you? Who is a genuine help during these difficult times? Again, treat yourself as you would treat a good friend and nurture yourself through these waves of emotion.

Before we end the chapter on anxiety, Jane has some important advice:

'Suffering from anxiety is horrible and it can be quite scary at times but it's really important to keep doing the things that matter to you, despite suffering from anxiety. Don't wait for the anxiety to go before you do the important things in life, do them anyway. Even if it feels scary. People's worlds can shrink when they stop doing the things they love because they are too terrified to do anything. Remember that you and your body have been through an awful lot to still be here and to still be alive. Given all that, you're allowed to want to live the best life that you can. And this means doing the things that are important to you. Keep in mind what matters to you and use that to drive you, rather than being driven by the anxiety'.

Top tip
Treat yourself with kindness and compassion when experiencing anxiety.

Checklist

Here's a recap of the key points for you to take away from this chapter.

There was a lot to take in from this chapter on anxiety! So, here's a recap of the key points and some more tips on how to calm your anxiety.

1 Understand that anxiety is a normal human reaction – these feelings and emotions that you're experiencing are a result of the threat

system in your brain working on overdrive. It's perfectly natural to be experiencing anxiety after the end of cancer treatment.

2 Learn to recognize what triggers your anxiety and how it manifests itself. What causes you to experience anxiety symptoms or to increase the anxiety? Is it reading about someone else's cancer experience? Is it having too much to do at work? Is it leaving the house to go somewhere new? Once you know the sorts of things that trigger your anxiety, you can work out how to cope with them with awareness.

3 When experiencing anxious symptoms, thank your brain and body for doing their job and for looking after you but note that you are okay and that you don't need the threat system to fire up at this moment.

4 Treat yourself with kindness and compassion – like you would treat a loved one or good friend.

5 Find ways of calming yourself. You could try:
   ○ breathing exercises
   ○ mindfulness exercises
   ○ meditation
   ○ going for a walk
   ○ yoga or Pilates
   ○ relaxing with your feet up
   ○ writing and journalling
   ○ drawing and painting
   ○ doing something active such as gardening, crafts, baking or reorganizing a cupboard
   ○ reading or listening to podcasts or audiobooks

6 The Toolkit at the back of the book provides guidance on breathing exercises, mindfulness exercises and journalling.

7 If you're experiencing anxious thoughts then don't fight them or push them down; instead, recognize that you're having such thoughts, thank your mind for trying to protect you, observe them and allow the thoughts to float away (using images of the thoughts floating away).

8 If you're feeling anxious, allow the feeling to arrive and breathe around it. You can try the exercise of imagining the emotion as a colour shape and breathing around that.

9   Don't stop yourself from doing the things that you love and which are important to you.

10 Try to avoid getting overwhelmed with life: take things slowly – there's no need to rush; don't feel an obligation to say yes to everything – it's okay to say no sometimes and understand that if you're suffering from fatigue, you might not be able to do everything that you used to do.

11 Keep yourself in the present by focusing what you are doing right here and now:
    ○ Stop what you're doing.
    ○ Take a few deep breaths.
    ○ Look around you.
    ○ Take note of everything that you can see.
    ○ Remind yourself that at this exact moment everything is fine. You are okay.

12 Consider taking a break from social media if you're feeling particularly anxious.

13 Take some time for yourself every day.

14 Exercise is known to help with anxiety, so try to incorporate exercise or activity into your daily routine. Only exercise at your level so if you're not used to exercising don't go for a long run. Things like gardening, house work, walking to the shops and taking the stairs not the lift are all good activities to get you started.

15 There is no shame in experiencing anxiety and if it's impacting your life on a day-to-day basis then you should seek help from a professional. Speak to your doctor or medical team as a starting point.

Notes

Use this page to process your anxiety in some of the ways that Jane has suggested

5

The fear of recurrence

Fearing that the cancer will return and adapting to the fact that there is no guarantee that the cancer won't come back

'When I was going through treatment, I found it easier to focus on the medical side of what I was going through rather than to try and process the emotional side of things. I like to focus on what I can control, and it was easier for me to focus on making my way through my medical plan than to get emotionally involved in what was happening. I celebrated the end of cancer treatment but after a couple of months I started to address what had just happened to me and I started to think about recurrence. Fear of recurrence is my biggest issue at the moment. I'm so worried that the cancer will come back. I feel that I need to be doing everything I can to stop it from coming back'.

Melissa

One of the major causes of anxiety after cancer treatment, is the fear that the cancer will return. Also known as THE FEAR. We all know that there is, sadly, no 100 per cent guarantee that cancer will not come back in the future. Yes, the medics will have given you the best possible treatment to help minimize the risk of the cancer coming back. But knowing that there is no guarantee that the cancer won't come back, can be particularly difficult and upsetting for many people to process. Mary has particularly struggled with the fear of a recurrence, and she told me:

'I know that my doctors have done their best to stop the cancer coming back, but I can't help wondering if it will. I question every ache and pain and anything that doesn't feel right in my body. I've never been like this before, but now I question every small change. I've got to the point where I'm convinced that I'll have cancer again and that I need to prepare for it. Cancer is still sitting on my shoulder, giving it a tap every now and again reminding me that it could come back'.

For those of you who've very recently completed cancer treatment, the fear of cancer returning can be particularly intense, after all, you've only just been through cancer and everything that it brings – such as a life-changing shock, intense stress, fear of dying, harsh treatment and unpleasant side-effects. Nobody – with such memories still fresh in their minds – wants to go through that again, and nobody wants to go one step further and be diagnosed with incurable cancer. But even if you finished treatment months or years ago, the fear of a cancer recurrence can still be with you, and for some of you this fear can impact you on a daily basis.

The impact upon daily life

Let's start by taking a look at the ways in which the fear of recurrence can impact daily life and first up is the way that this fear is all-consuming. It's there all day and all night. It can stop you from sleeping, it can prevent you from concentrating on work and it can hang over you as you're trying to do all the normal things with which you so desperately want to get on. I liken the fear to a little black cloud that's following you around all day and night dripping fear into your thoughts. It's there while you're emptying the dishwasher and trying to think of what to have for dinner. It's there while you're parking the car at the shops. It's there as you order your starter and main course at a friend's birthday dinner. It's there all the time. Sometimes it might feel like the cloud is releasing a relentless torrential downpour of fear into your head, whilst at other, calmer moments, it might feel like the dark cloud has drifted away for a little while, allowing you to momentarily clear your thoughts of fears.

Does this sound familiar? If so, you are most certainly not the only one feeling this way. For example, Gabi described what she was going through in this way:

> 'During treatment I put on a coat of armour and charged through: it was the only way I could cope. I knew that if a single chink developed in the armour, then I would completely crumble. When treatment ended and I went back to work, I found myself alone a lot of the time. It was at this point that the armour started to fall away – treatment had ended and I felt that I didn't need to keep my guard up so much. I was experiencing a lot of aches and pains – due to the hormone treatment I was taking following treatment – and I was convinced that the cancer was back. My mind was torturing me with the fear of a cancer recurrence'.

Mary and Kate also talked to me about their fear of recurrence. Mary said:

> 'I feel like I've convinced myself I will get cancer again. It's almost as if I have accepted it as the normal process to have cancer twice'.

And Kate explained:

> 'Every time I'm in the shower I always check for a breast lump. I'm reminded of my cancer and that it could return every time I look in the mirror and see the tattoo spots in my cleavage from radiation and every time, I go to shave my underarm and see my two scars from my lymph node removal. I don't think there is ever a day where I don't have that fear sitting somewhere in my head'.

In addition to the all-consuming nature of the fear of recurrence, there are triggers in day-to-day life that can cause you worry about a recurrence. Take all those twinges, aches and pains. Clearly, it's perfectly normal – and expected – to experience innocent aches and pains, but if you've just been through cancer, aches and pains are far from innocent. The usual thought process goes something like this...

What's that ache?
Is it cancer?
Is it a harmless ache that will just pass and disappear?
Is it cancer?
Is it normal?
Is it cancer?
Is it a lingering side-effect of treatment?
Is it cancer?
Is it a side-effect of the medication that I'm currently on?
Is it cancer?
It's cancer.

Kathryn understands this thought process and told me:

> 'Every time I feel a twinge in my body, I wonder whether I need to get it checked out'.

Jo H said that she felt the same way, and explained to me:

> 'I was getting some localized pain in my right breast that I was getting myself worked up about. I was convinced the cancer had come back'.

And Emily commented:

> 'If I get a headache or I don't feel well, my mind instantly goes to: what if it's cancer? It's such a big part of who I am now and I don't trust my body. I've had cancer once so what if I have it again? I'm trying to come to terms with this'.

Another way that this fear of recurrence can impact your life is the way that it can make you feel like you're living on borrowed time: there is sometimes the sense that you have a limited time before cancer comes back and you have to go through the trauma of treatment again or – in a worst-case scenario – that treatment might not be successful the next time.

Living with this feeling of borrowed time can give some people an impatient need to live their very best life right here and right now: an urge to travel the world, have life-changing experiences (good ones this time), and make wonderful memories. This can be invigorating and exciting for some people, like Mary who said:

'I have a feeling that I must live my life now in case cancer comes back. It's more important than ever for me to get married and start a family'.

But it can be stressful and overwhelming for others, like Kathryn, who told me:

'I want to fit in as much as possible with my daughter now because every moment that I'm not making memories or having experiences with her, is lost time that we may not get back should the cancer come back. I've found myself taking so many photos all the time because I was so worried that if the cancer came back, she wouldn't have long-term memories'.

Whilst the fear of recurrence can be particularly intense in the period shortly after the end of treatment, it can continue further down the line so that even at three- or thirteen-years post-treatment, there is still a fear. It is perfectly normal to continue to worry that the cancer might come back, after all there is always a risk. For example, Juliet is five years post-diagnosis and she explained:

'I don't think about recurrence unless I have an unexplained pain. The fear of recurrence has gradually subsided over time and it's helped me to remember that you shouldn't worry about things out of your control or which haven't happened'.

So, how do you process this lack of a guarantee that the cancer will not return? How do you manage the fear of cancer returning? Can it even be managed? To answer this last question, yes, it can be managed. But before we look at how to manage it, it's actually helpful to understand two things: firstly, that it's totally normal to be feeling this way, and secondly, why you feel this way. And we're going to look at all of this with help from Dr Jane Clark[1] again.

Fear of a recurrence is normal

First things first, Jane says that it's important to recognize that it is absolutely totally 100 per cent normal to worry about the recurrence of cancer. Moreover, it's important to recognize that it's also normal to become what you might call 'hypervigilant' about your body. This is all that worrying you're doing about those little niggles, aches and pains – worrying that any new or different feeling in your body is the cancer back again. People who've had cancer are highly likely to check their bodies more frequently for abnormalities, for example, women who've had breast cancer might be frequently checking their breasts and armpits looking for lumps. It's all perfectly normal.

Jane says that it's worth pointing out that the way you feel about a possible recurrence of cancer may be affected by how you found your cancer in the first place. Take someone whose cancer was found during a routine screening appointment. They might not have noticed anything different going on in their body and were it not for the screening appointment, the cancer may not have been found so early. Someone in this situation may well worry that they didn't even know the cancer was there in the first place and question how they'll know if it returns. On the other hand, take someone who noticed something abnormal in their body and took themselves off to their doctor to get it checked out only to be diagnosed with cancer as a result. Someone in this situation may be worried about coming across an abnormality again – the mere discovery of something like a breast lump again can sometimes scare someone from regularly checking.

Nonetheless, however your cancer was originally discovered, fearing a recurrence of the cancer is one of the most common challenges faced during – and beyond recovery.

Why am I feeling this way?

To help understand how to cope with the fear of a cancer recurrence, it's important to address why a fear of recurrence can induce such anxiety. Let's go back to the threat system and the smoke detector that Jane explained in the anxiety chapter (Chapter 4). Remember how your brain has an inbuilt threat system that automatically begins to react if it perceives you to be in danger? Well, worrying about the cancer coming back will trigger this threat system. You don't have any control over that.

And remember the faulty smoke detector? Well, the smoke detector is still going off intermittently and it's not returning to its usual vigilance mode. The smoke detector has already had to deal with one fire (your original cancer diagnosis) and even though there's no smoke now, it's still on hyper-alert because it knows that there could be another fire. It wants to keep you protected by being better safe than sorry.

Another key point to note here – in understanding why this fear has such a huge impact on you – is that the 'cost' of a cancer recurrence is perceived as very high. Let me explain: if an event were to cause minor problems, then it would have a 'low cost' which is to say that the anxiety relating to that 'low cost' event would be minimal. But with cancer, the 'cost' of recurrence could be high – I mean, at the most extreme, it could cost you your life – so the anxiety reaction is greater. It has a higher cost.

Experiencing anxiety due to the fear of a cancer recurrence is a normal reaction of the brain. The brain is just doing its job. In order to cope with the feelings associated with a fear of recurrence, the first step is dealing with the anxiety that this fear is producing.

How to manage the fear of recurrence

So, now that you know it's normal to have a fear of recurrence and why you're feeling this fear, the big question is how can you deal with the fear? Jane is here to help with this, and her first piece of advice is that it's really important to recognize that you can't switch off this fear. Unfortunately, you can't make it go away, so instead you need to work out how you can calm it and deal with it when it gets particularly intense. In order to understand this, it's time for another analogy from Jane. This is the flooding river analogy:[2]

> 'Think of yourself walking along a path next to a river. When you're diagnosed with cancer the river rises, completely flooding your path and causing cata- strophic damage to everything on the path. All you can do at the moment of the flood is to deal with the flood water. Your hands are completely full dealing with the immediate crisis of the flood – the cancer diagnosis. But in time – as you go through cancer treatment – the flood water gradually recedes. Nevertheless, it takes every ounce of strength and all your resilience to deal with the flood and help the water recede.

Once the water level of the river has returned to normal – when treatment is over – you're left with a path that's been badly damaged by the flood. Everything on the path that you're now standing on, and ahead of you as far as you can see, has been damaged by the flood. So now you're tasked with rebuilding the path. You have to decide in which direction to build the path. You need to consider what might help you to rebuild the path: what tools you need and how to go about it.

Whilst rebuilding the path, you continue to walk along it and guess what ... the river is still there, right next to the path. You know that at any time, the river could suddenly flood the path again – a cancer recurrence – and you know that if it did that again you'd be unable to do anything other than deal with the immediate crisis of the flood. In fact, anyone walking along the path who hasn't had cancer isn't even aware that the river could unexpectedly flood. But you know that it could flood at any time and that you can't do anything to prevent it.

As you're walking along the path you can hear the river. Sometimes it's a loud rushing sound at which point you're much more aware of, and worried about, the danger of possible flooding. At other times you might not even hear the river and you can walk along the path without thinking about the possibility of a flood.

Sometimes, you're so worried about another flood that, rather than continuing along the path, you find yourself standing and staring at the river looking for signs of the water rising. But if you do that, then you're missing out on what's on the path ahead (your life ahead of you)'.

So, how can you move along the path knowing that the river is right there, that you can't get away from the river and that you have no control over the possibility of a flood? How do you monitor the risk of another flood whilst continuing your journey along the path? The challenge is to learn to live alongside the river knowing the river is always going to be there. But there are things that can help. Think about some flood management systems that might be in place: your hospital has a flood management system – for example, your monitoring scans and appointments – and you can implement your own flood management system by being vigilant about abnormal changes and knowing when to get them checked out. You can also make plans for those days when the river is really noisy. It might be particularly noisy if you have an upcoming scan, or if you've read of a celebrity being diagnosed with the type of cancer that you had or if cancer is in the media because it's an awareness month.

The key is to find ways to live alongside this river, ways to help yourself when the river gets particularly loud and ways to make your path what you really want it to be. Think about what really matters to you and how you can make your path in life reflect that. You, more than anyone, know that we don't get a second shot at life so how can you make this the life you want to lead?

Everyone is different and people will find different coping mechanisms that suit them. Here are Jane's suggestions to get you started:

- When you feel anxious about recurrence, don't dismiss it and berate yourself for feeling this way. Understand that anxiety is perfectly normal and you need to treat yourself with kindness and compassion. Take a look at the chapter on anxiety (Chapter 4) for advice on dealing with anxiety.
- Think about the impact of social media on your fear of recurrence. Do you follow and read the stories of people who have had cancer recurrence or a spread of their cancer? How does it make you feel to read what these people say on social media? Be aware that doing this might increase your anxiety rather than give you any benefit. Everyone is different in how they react to other people's stories, just make sure that you are doing what's best for you.
- There are lots of support groups where you can talk about your fear of recurrence with other people who are feeling the same way as you. It's worth looking for specific groups that deal with moving on and living with the uncertainty after cancer. The Useful Resources section at the back of the book has details of some national charities but it is also worth asking your medical team to refer you to local groups.
- Dealing with uncertainty can lead people to doing things where they feel like they are taking control. For example, changing their diets and lifestyle. This is the brain's normal way of working in uncertain situations: it's looking for a sense of control. Whilst it is good to be making healthy choices about what you eat and how you live your life, it's important to maintain a balance and not go over the top in trying to establish control because that in itself can also cause anxiety. For example, some people may give up sugar. For some, giving up sugar might be the best thing they've ever done and they thrive in their sugar-free world. For others though, it can make them miserable because firstly it's torture for them not to have anything sweet ever, but also because if they do then have a piece of cake, they feel terribly

guilty for days thereafter. Everyone is different and it's important to work out what's best for you.

Turning to those annoying aches, pains and twinges now; there are some specific ways to deal with all the worry about every ache, pain, niggle or anything abnormal going on with your body. Here's Jane's advice:

- Remember that before you had cancer, just as now, you didn't have any certainty about your health. So how did you work out if you needed to see a doctor about something back then? You probably had a subconscious list of rules that you followed when assessing if, and when, you needed to see a doctor. This would have included things like the intensity of a pain and the length of time you were experiencing a symptom. So, why not draw up some new ground rules for getting things checked out, including the quantifiable things to monitor. Family doctors, oncologists and oncology nurses can help advise you on this – they're very experienced at knowing at which point to get something checked out.

- The fear of recurrence can be particularly intense in the middle of the night. We've all been there – it's then that you can find yourself going on a little journey on the mind train into the future, thinking the worst. Let's say you're awake in the middle of the night and you can't sleep because you have a back ache that's been bothering you for a few days. Rather than putting the back ache down to the Zumba class you did a few days ago, you're probably lying there thinking that the cancer is back and that it's spread to your spine. As you lie there in the dark, you can picture telling the doctor about the back ache and, given your history, you see the doctor's face falling as they send you off for a scan. You'll imagine going for the scan, and you might even start working out if you'll be able to take the time off work and who will collect the children from school while you're at the hospital. You'll visualize sitting in the hospital chair, being told that it's cancer and how you'll feel. You'll picture telling your family and their reaction. And on and on and on. You'll see all of this happening as if it's all real and happening right then and there. The mind can be so powerful that, lying there in the middle of the night, you'll start believing that this little journey is the truth. The key here is to recognize right at the start of this little thought train, that your mind is going off on a little fictional journey and that you need to bring it back to the here and now.

- If your mind goes on a little journey, getting ahead of itself, and you need to bring it back to the here and now a helpful way is to tell yourself that you don't need to deal with those future situations (the doctor's appointment, the scan, the scan results, the diagnosis and the treatment), right now but *if* you ever need to, you will be able to do so. Recognize that you will deal with all of those situations in due course if and when needed, but recognize that right now there are other explanations for the back ache. Go back to your ground rules for getting aches and pains checked out.

- If you're worried about a particular ache or pain, for example a headache, try listing all the other reasons why you might have a headache. It could be down to eye strain, feeling stressed, tense muscles, being dehydrated, just a random headache and so on. Now, you could try allocating a percentage possibility against each of these, up to a total of 100 per cent. For example, you might think that there is a 50 per cent chance that the headache is down to dehydration as you haven't drunk much water today; there's a 30 per cent chance that it's eye-strain as you've been working at your laptop for the whole day without taking many breaks; and there's a 20 per cent chance it's tense muscles because work is pretty stressful today. So, this leaves a 10 per cent chance of the headache being something else, let alone being cancer. The more reasonable alternative explanations for the headache, the less percentage chance of the headache being a sign of cancer recurrence.

- When you're feeling particularly anxious about an ache or pain, it can help to talk it over with someone who will help you look at the situation rationally and not from a point of panic. It's important to pick the right person for this. Don't pick your over-vigilant, hyper-cautious friend who'll drag you down to the hospital before you've even finished describing the symptoms. And don't pick the dismissive friend or family member who'll brush off your concerns almost as soon as you start talking about them. People who haven't had cancer can (although not always) be dismissive about these sorts of worries, and it's easy to not feel heard by friends and family when you talk to them about your fears. It's important that you feel that you are heard – after all, your fears are rational. Talk to a sensible, rational person, whether that's a friend, family member or one of your medical team like the oncology nurse. If you have a breast care nurse, for example, they are very experienced in talking about these sorts of situations and even though you might feel that you don't want to disturb them/take up their valuable time/be seen as an over-worrier this is all part of their job and they are very good at it. So, don't hesitate to call them.

- Don't dismiss your concerns and fears yourself. It's very easy to tell yourself not to be so silly and that you should pull yourself together and stop worrying. Understand it is a serious worry and that you need to be compassionate and kind to yourself.

- Human brains don't like uncertainty or grey areas. They like certainty. When you have a grey area of uncertainty, your brain will naturally try to solve it. Let me give you an example: you've been for a scan about a shoulder pain and while you're waiting for the results your brain will naturally try to solve the issue because it doesn't like being in a state of uncertainty. So, you'll probably start thinking things like, if the scan results show cancer, then I'll have to go and see the oncologist and then I'll need to tell my family and then I'll need to tell my friends but maybe this time I won't tell everyone and then I'll need to sort out some time off work because I'll probably need surgery and on and on … You're back on that mind train again. Your brain is trying to solve an uncertain issue. Your brain can't help it. Be aware that this is a natural way for the brain to work. Bring yourself back to the present – our only certainty is today and so bring yourself back to the here and now. Don't think too far ahead – you don't need the planning and organizing part of the brain to get involved in this situation because you just don't know what is ahead of you. Be kind and patient with yourself.

- Mindfulness can help bring yourself back to the present. There are mindfulness exercises and breathing exercises in the Toolkit at the back of the book but here's a quick exercise that you can do at any time of day or night, wherever you are:
  - Put your feet hip distance apart of the floor, feel the ground beneath your feet.
  - Put your hand gently on your stomach.
  - Close your eyes.
  - Take five breaths in and out.

○ Bring yourself back to the present and think about what you can see, hear, touch, smell and taste right now.

○ Remind yourself that you're present in the here and now and you're okay right at this minute.

The signs and symptoms of a recurrence

Part of the fear about a cancer recurrence can be down to the fact that you know there's a risk, but you don't know much about the risk. You may, or may not, have been told by your oncologist about the risks and signs of your cancer coming back as a recurrence or as secondary cancer. If you haven't been told, then it's worth educating yourself.

With insight and advice from Dr Sophie McGrath (the Breast Cancer Oncologist to whom I've already introduced you to back in Chapter 2), the remainder of this chapter talks about the ways in which breast cancer can come back, together with the signs and symptoms. This might sound like a scary thing to read about, but remember that fear is sometimes fear of the unknown. If you're not up to thinking about this today, perhaps you could bookmark this section to read at a later date.

The first thing to understand is that there are three different types of recurrence that can occur. In relation to breast cancer, you could experience one or more of the following:

- A local cancer recurrence which is where breast cancer returns in close proximity to the location of the original tumour.
- Secondary cancer (also known as advanced breast cancer, stage four breast cancer and metastatic breast cancer) which is where breast cancer cells have spread from the original tumour to other organs of the body: the bones, liver, brain, lungs and/or skin.
- A new incidence of primary breast cancer which is not strictly a 'recurrence' because it's a new cancer in another part of the same breast as the original tumour or in the other breast.

Let's park the issue of secondary breast cancer for a moment and take the first and third of these possible recurrences to begin with: a local recurrence and a new incidence of primary breast cancer. You're probably well aware of the signs of breast cancer by now – seeing as you've just had it – but there's no harm in reminding yourself. This is especially important if your breast cancer was found by a routine mammogram rather than by yourself.

Remember that you need to keep an eye on the entire chest area – including the armpits and collarbone area – and not just where your original breast cancer originated. It's important to check your breasts and chest area regularly, but not obsessively. It might be tempting to check your breasts every day in the shower, but that isn't necessary and it will just cause you stress. Regular monitoring is doing a full check once or twice a month, whilst being aware of obvious changes in between checks. So, keep an eye open for:

- a new lump or thickening in your breast, collarbone or armpit
- a change in size, shape or feel of your breast
- skin changes in the breast such as puckering, dimpling, a rash or redness of the skin
- fluid leaking from the nipple (in women who aren't pregnant or breastfeeding)
- changes in the position of the nipple.

There are various places where you can find advice on checking your breasts and I've included a list of helpful charities in the Useful Resources section at the back of the book.

Remember that if you find anything of concern, don't panic because sometimes your breasts change after cancer treatment and a new lump might be down to fat necrosis, scarring or a benign cyst. However, if you do notice any changes, it's super important to always get in touch with your medical team, breast care nurse or doctor so you can get it checked out properly. It might be scary to do this, but it's important to have a professional check out what is going on.

Now let's turn to the topic of secondary breast cancer. You may not have heard about secondary breast cancer before you were diagnosed with primary breast cancer – I certainly hadn't. In fact, it's quite common for someone who hasn't been impacted by breast cancer to just assume that there is one type of breast cancer, as opposed to the various different types, grades and stages of breast cancer. Even if you've just been through breast cancer treatment, you may still not have heard about secondary breast cancer. Being told about the signs and symptoms of secondary breast cancer may or may not be routine for your hospital. Not all oncologists, oncology teams or nurses provide this information to patients at the end of treatment for primary breast cancer. It's a difficult balancing act for the medical team: on the one hand it's important for a patient to be fully informed so that they can be self-aware, but on the other hand it's a very scary thing for a patient to suddenly be faced with after everything they've just been through. In fact, it's perfectly possible that you might be getting worried and feeling overwhelmed whilst reading this section of the book, in which case why don't you have a warm drink, take a break, maybe do a breathing exercise from the Toolkit at the back of the book and then revisit this topic in a little while.

To start the discussion on the topic of secondary breast cancer, Dr Sophie McGrath is going to explain what it is and refer to a few statistics.

Secondary breast cancer is stage four breast cancer and it's also known as 'advanced' breast cancer or 'metastatic' breast cancer. In those people with a history of early – primary – breast cancer, medics and scientists think that some of the breast cancer cells can sometimes remain 'sleeping' in the blood or lymphatic system and then – at some point in the future – wake up and spread to other parts of the body (most commonly the liver, lungs, brain, skin and bones) despite previous treatment to try to prevent this happening.

As at the time of writing this book, roughly five in every one hundred people with breast cancer already have secondaries when their cancer is first diagnosed (which is termed 'de novo' secondary breast cancer)[3] and some people who've had primary breast cancer go on to develop secondary breast cancer a number of years after their primary diagnosis. It is estimated that around 35,000 people are currently living with secondary breast cancer in the UK[4]. Sadly, there is currently no cure for secondary breast cancer. Depending on a number of factors – including the particular type of breast cancer, how far the cancer has spread, where it has spread to and for how long the cancer has been spreading – the length of time that someone can survive after a diagnosis of secondary breast cancer varies greatly (up to a number of years) and its spread can often (but not always) be controlled with treatments.

When it comes to secondary breast cancer, the signs and symptoms are different to those of primary breast cancer. The Useful Resources at the back of the book has a helpful infographic showing the signs and symptoms of secondary breast cancer so please go and have a read of that. Familiarize yourself with these signs and symptoms and talk to your medical team about them.

Now that you know the signs and symptoms to be looking out for, some of you might want to know your own personal risks of getting a recurrence or secondary breast cancer. This is totally individual and some of you are probably reading this thinking that there is no way you want to know this! However, if you think you would like to know your personal risk, this is where it's very important to talk to your oncologist. It is possible for your oncologist to get an idea of your chances of surviving the next five, ten and fifteen years from the NHS Predict Tool that we discussed in Chapter 2. This is big decision to make, and you shouldn't make it lightly. If you're considering asking your oncologist for the statistics applicable to you, please refer back to the words of caution in Chapter 2. Furthermore, I've got three warnings for you:

1 Remember that trying to make sense of statistics can be tricky and they might be difficult for you to get your head around.
2 Remember that once you've heard a statistic, you can't unhear it.
3 Remember that statistics (including any statistics relating to your personal risks) are a guide and can be wrong.

When it comes to monitoring your health for signs and symptoms of a cancer recurrence, I've got three final pieces of advice:

1 Trust your instincts. It's very important to get to know your body and what's normal for you. Insist on check-ups and scans when you feel that something isn't right. You know your body better than anyone else. Don't be embarrassed to make an appointment if you're worried about something.
2 Avoid the internet (and Dr Google). It's not a good idea to use the internet to research information about cancer recurrences and secondary cancer risks. Instead, ask your medical team your questions and to find out more information, look at reputable cancer charity websites. There's a list of helpful websites in the Useful Resources section at the back of the book.
3 Always get professional medical advice. Always ask your breast surgeon, oncologist, breast care nurse or medical team about anything that is worrying you. Don't be afraid or embarrassed to ask ANYTHING and as helpful as the cancer community on social media is, don't rely on social media for medical advice.

> **Top tip**
> When you find yourself going on a little mind journey, thinking about the what-ifs and worst-case scenarios, bring yourself back to the here and now.

Checklist

Here's a recap of the key points for you to take away from this chapter

1 Understand that experiencing the what-if wobbles and worrying about cancer coming back is entirely normal for anyone who's had cancer and it's a normal reaction of the brain.

2 Know that you can't switch off this fear, but you can learn ways to calm it and deal with it.

3 Don't berate yourself for feeling this way: treat yourself with kindness and compassion.

4 Get to know what triggers bouts of fear of recurrence. If reading about other people's experiences on social media triggers the fear for you, consider avoiding these accounts and maybe spend less time on social media.

5 Find a local support group, or online support group, where you can talk to other people who are feeling the same way as you.

6 Know that all aches and pains do not mean the cancer has returned: remember that before you had cancer, you would have had all sorts of aches and pains.

7 If you're worried about an ache or pain, use the percentage possibility tool to remind yourself of the minimal chances of it being cancer.

8 Educate yourself on the ways that cancer may return: it could be a local recurrence, secondary breast cancer or a new incidence of breast cancer.

9 Make sure you know how to properly check your breasts for signs of cancer, and perform regular – but not obsessive – checks.

10 Familiarize yourself with the signs of secondary cancer. There is a section in the Useful Resources on the signs and symptoms of secondary breast cancer.

11 Trust your instincts. Get to know your body and what is normal for you. Insist on check-ups and scans when you feel that something

isn't right. Don't let anyone make you feel like a hypochondriac. You know your body better than anyone else. Don't be embarrassed to make an appointment if you are worried about something.

12 Always get professional medical advice if you're worried about anything. Always ask your surgeon, oncologist, nurse or medical team about anything that is worrying you. Don't be afraid or embarrassed to ask anything.

13 Watch out for unhelpful thoughts – you can't control what's going to happen so don't waste your energy worrying about it. Keep grounded in the here and now. The Toolkit at the back of the book has some helpful mindfulness and breathing exercises to help you bring yourself back to the present when you find yourself thinking about the uncertain future.

14 Live your life and enjoy every day! Despite the risks of recurrence and secondary cancer, don't let it take over your life.

Notes

Use this page to make notes on what you've learnt about coping with the fear of recurrence

6

Why me?

Questioning why you got cancer

'I do ask "why me?" I was really healthy: I'm young, I don't smoke, I was fit and exercised a lot – I was an athlete. It doesn't make sense to my logical brain: it feels so out of control and I don't like feeling out of control'.

Jo L

As you've probably noticed by now, this period at the end of cancer treatment is often the time when you start to really think about what you've been through. You may not have had the time, energy or brain space to process your cancer diagnosis properly while going through treatment. After all, you were probably focusing on getting through some fairly harsh treatment. So, it's perfectly normal that now – after treatment – you begin to process everything. And as you process what you've just been through, it's not uncommon to ask yourself questions such as:

- Why me?
- Why did I get cancer?
- What did I do wrong?
- What didn't I do right?
- What should I have eaten/drunk/done to have prevented getting cancer?

If you've had cancer, it's entirely natural to want to know why you got it and what you didn't do right, so that you can make sense of what you've just been through and make sure that it doesn't happen again. The issue of why I got breast cancer used to keep me awake at night. I just couldn't understand why, at the age of 42, breast cancer came knocking at my door. I'd followed the rules: I'd done everything I should have done to avoid ever getting cancer. For goodness sake, I'd drunk green tea and kale smoothies for years. What did I do wrong?

Some of you might have these sorts of questions running around continually in your head, whilst some of you might only think about it every now and again. Wondering *why me?* can creep up on you when you're not expecting it – something might trigger the question and surrounding emotions, such as reaching an anniversary of your diagnosis, or learning of someone else's diagnosis.

So, what's the answer to question, *why me?* Well, there isn't a straight-forward answer and, actually working out why you got cancer is a complicated business which is impacted by a number of factors that you can't control. According to Dr Sophie McGrath (remember the oncologist to whom I introduced you a few chapters back?) it may involve your genes, your lifestyle, your emotional well-being, the various systems within your body and much, much more. Whilst it's known that there are genes which can increase your chance of getting some types of cancer (for example the BRCA gene and its relationship to breast cancer) and that certain lifestyles can increase or decrease the risk of developing cancer, it's important to remember that even if you live a healthy lifestyle and tick all the boxes on the 'what to do to prevent getting cancer' check-list, there is still a chance of getting cancer.

Sophie says that alterations can occur in the genes within cells causing cells to mutate. Sometimes these mutations are just not caught by the body's defence system. So, sadly, at the end of the day, getting cancer is often down to a random combination of factors. That's all. Don't blame yourself for having had cancer. It's not your fault. At the time of writing this book, the statistics are that there's a one in two chance of getting cancer.[1] Sadly, you've been the one in that two.

I know it's all very well being told these scientific facts, but you're probably wondering how knowing these facts actually helps you to process the *why me?* question. Barbara Babcock, Coach and Trainee Family Therapist, is here to help us again (she helped us back in Chapter 3 on the issues of the safety-net and lack of purpose). Barbara suggests that to start with, rather than looking at what you didn't do right, maybe think of your diagnosis as a random event. She likens a cancer diagnosis to unfortunately drawing the winning ticket in a lottery you didn't know you'd entered (and that you wouldn't have wanted to play if you'd known). And, as Barbara recognizes, the trouble with getting to grips with the randomness of your diagnosis is the fact that the human brain likes certainty and doesn't like uncertainty. Unfortunately, being unable to answer the *why me?* question creates a big juicy chunk of uncertainty in your brain, and it is often this uncertainty which is contributing to a lot of the unease that you're feeling.

So, with Barbara's help, let's go back to the *why me?* question and break it down. She says that it can be helpful if you consider the reasons why you're asking the question. Are you asking *why me?* because you're angry? Or sad? Or grieving? If you can identify the feeling or feelings behind the question, then you can address those feelings in a safe way with kindness and compassion.

As you all know, these feelings of anger, sadness and grief are often stigmatized in our society but they are a normal part of being human and a natural part of the cancer experience. To move beyond these feelings, you'll need to process them, and Barbara's advice is that it's best to not try to push the feelings back down inside you because by doing that, you risk them leaking out and making you feel even worse. She suggests that if you're feeling overwhelmed by these feelings then it would be helpful to process them with a therapist, counsellor or coach. If you're feeling up to exploring these feelings on your own, then here are Barbara's tips:

- Allow yourself to sit and think about these feelings for a couple of minutes – maybe set a timer – after which try to get on with something completely different. It might take a few of these two-minute sessions over a period of time to move forward, but by doing this you're acknowledging the feelings and allowing them to move on. You could also use these two-minute sessions to draw your feelings or write about them (perhaps use the notes page at the end of this chapter).
- Sometimes it helps to reframe the question from *why me?* to *why not me?* For some people, looking at the question this way will open up other ways of understanding.
- Talking to a professional can help. As this person is not personally invested in you or your future, they are in a good position to help you find your own path.
- Writing and journalling can be a huge help in exploring your feelings. By writing your feelings onto a piece of paper you allow the page to hold the heaviness of your feelings rather than the heaviness sitting within you. You can take all the spinning, jumbling thoughts and put them on paper in order to make sense of them and thus how you're feeling. Things to think about when writing and journalling are:

○ When you consider the question, *why me?* what thoughts are you having? Write down these thoughts.

○ What are you feeling? Sadness? Anger? Grief? Fear? Something else? Notice where you feel those feelings in your body – are they in your stomach, chest, a weight on your shoulders, a tight neck or somewhere else? Sit with the body sensations for a little while. Notice how they change and write about the sensations.

○ Sometimes, the *why me?* question relates to feelings of loss resulting from cancer. Loss of, for example, certainty, a relationship, a favourite activity you can no longer do, physical energy, or spontaneity. Note down what you feel you have lost. If these losses were things that you very much valued, allow yourself to mourn them. Also note down what you have gained, newfound strength and resilience, new friends, a greater appreciation for life and so on. How might you use and celebrate these gains? Chapter 12 looks at loss and grief in more detail and provides some guidance on coping with these emotions.

○ Think about how someone you trust, who has been through a similar experience to you, would advise you on dealing with the *why me?* question. Try writing down what they would say to you.

○ If writing isn't your thing, it's possible to connect with thoughts and feelings around your cancer experience in other ways such as drawing, painting, sculpting, crafting, exercise/sport, cooking, baking, singing, knitting, woodworking and so on. There really is something for everyone, it's just a question of finding the thing that works for you.

• The *why me?* question can feel like a struggle. What would happen if you put the struggle to one side for a moment? What are you noticing now? How could you use your energy which was focused on the struggle but is now freed up?

• Talking to an understanding partner, spouse, friend, family member or peer with a similar experience can help. By talking to someone about your feelings, that person will share the heaviness of your feelings allowing you to feel lighter. You might be worried about being a burden to these people if you take your feelings to them. But don't. You're not the burden. The problem – the feelings – are the burden and kind compassionate friends and family will allow you to share the burden with them.

> **Top tip**
> Try to work out what emotions are going on behind the question of why you got cancer.

Checklist

Here's a recap of the key points for you to take away from this chapter.

1 It's perfectly normal to question why you got cancer.
2 Understand that whilst your genes and lifestyle can impact a risk of cancer, it's often a random event.
3 Consider why you're asking this question. Is there another emotion behind the question such as anger, sadness or grief? Some of the feelings behind the question are dealt with in other chapters such as loss and grief (Chapter 12) and anxiety (Chapter 4).
4 It can be helpful to use writing and journalling to explore your feelings around this question. The Toolkit at the back of the book contains some writing prompts, but prompts specific to this question could be:
   ○ I feel sad that ...
   ○ I feel angry that ...
   ○ I fear that ...
   ○ I have lost ...
   ○ I have gained ...
5 It can help to reframe the question to *why not me?* instead of *why me?*
6 Talking about how you feel can help you to process this question. You could talk to a good friend, a charity helpline or seek professional counselling.

Notes

Use this page to answer some of the writing prompts in exploring the *Why me?* question.

7

Flashbacks and post-traumatic stress reactions

A traumatic event can be defined as a very extreme event during which you believe that you might die

'For a time after treatment ended, I would find myself flashing back to certain situations from my treatment – times when I was particularly scared like when I was diagnosed, my first chemotherapy infusion and when I was in intensive care. These would happen out of the blue if I was doing something where my mind wandered. They've calmed down now and I tend to only get them if something specific triggers the memory'.

Cathy

As you've probably gathered by now, there are many complex emotions and feelings that can materialize at the point of completing cancer treatment, some of which can last for a number of years. And the subject of this chapter is yet another example ... flashbacks.

Flashbacks are when you feel as if you are right back in a specific time and situation again. Hands up who's gone to hospital for a routine appointment since finishing treatment, and experienced a flashback to the point at which you were diagnosed, or to the time you were really ill after chemotherapy, or to the day you heard that your scan results showed a spread to the lymph nodes? And with the flashback, hands up who also experienced an accompanying fear, anxiety and/or physical reaction such as shaking, sweating, feeling on edge, irritability, racing thoughts, nausea, and difficulty concentrating?

Both Kathryn and Molly experienced flashbacks for a while after the end of treatment. Kathryn told me:

'I get a lot of flashbacks at night: I'm back in the room where I was told I had cancer and I feel the same fear of dying that I felt then'.

And Molly explained:

> 'When I had my second zoledronic acid infusion a couple weeks ago on the cancer ward, I had a panic attack. I was definitely experiencing trauma due to being back in the cancer ward where I was hearing all the familiar noises, seeing the cold cap machines, seeing the other women leaving chemo and my heart breaking as I remembered how horrendous I would feel after treatment'.

According to Dr Jane Clark (the Consultant Clinical Psychologist who has provided insights and advice on a number of challenges in the book) it's perfectly normal to have flashbacks to times and events from during your diagnosis and treatment. She notes that the intensity of these flashbacks will differ from person to person and not everyone who has had cancer will have them. If this is something that you have experienced, or are continuing to experience, then read on to understand:

- What is a flashback?
- Why might someone experience a flashback?
- Why do the flashbacks come after the end of treatment?
- What triggers the flashbacks?
- How do you process the trauma that is causing the flashbacks?

What is a flashback?

To start with, according to Jane, when people talk about experiencing flashbacks it's likely that the person is experiencing something termed, in the psychological world, a 'post-traumatic stress reaction'. This essentially means that they've been through a traumatic, out of the ordinary experience, and their brain is still trying to make sense of it. They have experienced trauma. So, in order to understand flashbacks, and how you can deal with them, it's necessary to first understand a little bit about *trauma*.

Jane explains trauma as an emotional response to events which create an overwhelming amount of stress. Trauma relates back to a traumatic event that you have experienced in the past – whether the recent past or from a long time ago. A traumatic event is a very extreme event during which you genuinely believed that you (or someone else) might die or have a serious injury, for example being in a car crash, fighting in a war or – guess what – being diagnosed with cancer.

With cancer, it's not just the actual diagnosis which is traumatic, but other life-threatening incidents throughout treatment can also be classed as traumatic events. For example, having a serious allergic reaction to a chemo drug, being told that the cancer is more serious than first thought or being hospitalized for a serious infection. Any time you feel like your life is at risk, you are experiencing a traumatic event. There can also be what psychologists call 'small t' traumas. These aren't necessarily times when you feel a threat to your life, but your sense of self is threatened – such as points where you feel humiliated, powerless or ashamed. So, as you can see, it's not uncommon to experience trauma as a result of having had cancer.

Why might someone experience a flashback?

Okay, so that explains why someone experiences trauma as a result of a cancer diagnosis, but *why* does someone experience flashbacks? According to Jane, simply put, having a flashback is your brain's way of trying to process and make sense of the trauma.

Why do flashbacks happen after treatment has finished?

But why does this happen? Why do you experience flashbacks *after* the end of treatment? Surely once treatment is over, the trauma is over? Jane explains that although the traumatic events are over, the memory of the trauma isn't over – and it's often only at this point that your brain actually starts to process it all. Remember, a flashback is your brain trying to process your trauma. And it's often at this point, once the immediate threat is over (now that all the treatment is over and you no longer have cancer), that your brain is finally able to process the trauma. This all sounds a bit complicated so let's take it one step at a time and put this into the context of your diagnosis and treatment.

The chances are that almost as soon as you'd received your diagnosis, you probably found yourself on a conveyor belt of treatment: going to hospital to get your blood tests, going to scans, having your surgery, recovering from surgery, having chemotherapy and on and on and on. Your focus during your treatment would have been all about going to hospital for a test, scan, check-up or treatment; or recovering from the last treatment and getting yourself ready for the next. Your focus will have been on physically getting through treatment and as a result you may not have had the time or the brain space to process the emotional trauma that you were experiencing.

However, since your treatment came to an end and you stepped off the conveyor belt of treatment, you now have more time on your hands and you don't need to constantly think about things like getting to hospital for a blood test, avoiding infections whilst your neutrophils are low or what you'll need to ask at your next oncology appointment. With the combination of less focus on treatment and more time to think, your mind is able to recognize that the imminent danger is over and feel safe enough to try to process the trauma of what you've been through.

What can trigger a flashback?

Okay, that explains a lot, but what triggers these flashbacks? Back to Jane ... She explains that flashbacks can be triggered by the sights, smells and sounds that your brain associates with the memory of your trauma. For example, sitting in the same waiting room you sat in immediately after getting your diagnosis could take you back to the point at which you heard the words, 'You've got cancer'. Smelling the distinctive chemo ward scent could take you back to a chemo appointment when you experienced a serious allergic reaction. Or, seeing one of the chemo ward nurses could trigger the trauma of going through treatment all the while not knowing if you'd make it out the other side.

It's time for another quick biology lesson from Jane – but stick with it because this is very interesting and it helps explain exactly what is going on in your brain to cause it to flashback.

The brain's primary purpose is to help you to survive, and therefore it needs to learn quickly if certain situations are life-threatening. If you return to a location where you experienced one of these perceived life-threatening events – such as where you received your cancer diagnosis – your brain will fire off signals to remind you that this is where something terrible happened. This is the flashback and this is why you may experience a strong desire to escape certain places in the hospital. By doing this, your brain is trying its best to keep you safe and keep you alive.

The part of the brain that sets off the threat response is the limbic system. However, there is a more rational part of your brain – the prefrontal cortex that we learnt about in Chapter 4 – which is trying to take charge of your behaviour and calm your body down. This part of the brain knows that although the hospital is associated with scary things, it's also the place that can make you better.

So, you need the logical and rational part of the brain – the prefrontal cortex – to help calm the part of the brain that is focused on survival and remembering the dangerous things by flashing back to them – the limbic system. You have to use your prefrontal cortex to teach the limbic system that its belief that the hospital is a dangerous place is out of date. The limbic system needs to be taught that although you were diagnosed with cancer and that going through treatment was a terrifying event, you survived and your life is no longer in danger. This is what is meant by *processing the trauma*. In practice, to stop the flashbacks, you have to help your brain to process the trauma.

That's a lot to take in. But understanding why you're experiencing flashbacks can help you to process your trauma which in turn will help to stop the flashbacks.

How do you process the trauma that is causing the flashbacks?

Okay, so processing the trauma means calming the part of your brain that is responsible for giving you the flashbacks. But how can you do that? According to Jane, the key here is to reduce the rawness and emotional intensity of the trauma memory.

Jane's advice is that you can do this by going over and over the memory – by talking about it or writing about it – to the point that you almost become bored by the memory. The aim is to get to the point where you no longer associate overwhelming anxiety with the memory and you can recognize that although something terrible happened causing a complete sea change in your life, you're now able to move forward. The aim is to remove the life-threatening aspect of the memory so that you can acknowledge that whilst it was an awful experience, you are safe now, you have the rest of your life ahead of you and it's safe to move on. This might all sound a bit scary – after all, not everyone wants to write or talk about that they've been through – so to help you through this, here are some practical tips from Jane:

- Talk about what happened to you. Talk about it a lot and talk to a variety of people. Talk about the trauma and what you've been through until the memory of your experience loses its intensity.
- Whilst it's helpful and supportive to talk to a professional therapist or counsellor, if this isn't possible for you then you can talk to other people. Talk to friends and family. Talk to people in a support group. Join Facebook groups and online forums for your type of cancer where you can talk to people who've been through the same experience as you. Find people in your position on social media to whom you can connect and talk about your experiences. Call one of the cancer charity helplines. The Useful Resources section at the back of the book lists places where you can find support groups.
- There is evidence that writing about a traumatic experience can also help minimize the emotional intensity of it and allow you to process the event in a similar way to talking about it. The Toolkit at the back of the book can get you started with writing about your trauma. And you can use the Notes page at the end of this chapter to start making some notes.
- If you are experiencing flashbacks to a certain hospital ward that you've not visited since being unwell there, it can be helpful to go and visit that ward. Again, the idea is to update the memory to say that although you once felt terrible there, you are now safe and well and returning as a visitor. Talk to your hospital team if you think something like this might help.
- If you are experiencing such debilitating effects from the traumatic reaction that you can't sleep or function day-to-day, talk to your hospital team about a referral to a specialist (such as a clinical psychologist) as there are effective evidence-based treatments to help with trauma reactions.

It's worth just pointing out that trauma is different to anxiety: Jane explains that trauma is a stuck memory from the past which carries a high emotional intensity, whereas anxiety is a state of mind focused more about the present and the future (than the past). It's important to flag this up because it's helpful to understand a bit about the emotions and feelings that you're experiencing and consequently what you can do to help deal with these emotions and feelings. The way in which you deal with trauma is slightly different to the way in which you deal with anxiety.

> **Top tip**
> Talking about what you've been through until it becomes almost boring to you, will help to minimize the emotional intensity of a traumatic memory and help reduce the flashbacks.

Checklist

Here's a recap of the key points for you to take away from this chapter

1 Understand that it's normal to experience flashbacks after a cancer diagnosis. There's nothing wrong with you – your brain is just doing its job.
2 Know that a flashback is the brain's way of starting to process the trauma that you have been through. In this case, the trauma will be the time, or times, during your diagnosis and treatment when you believed that you might die.
3 It's important to understand that it's not unusual to experience this type of flashback after the end of treatment and to recognize that it's a sign from your brain that there is a trauma that needs processing. A flashback to a traumatic event is a sign that your brain hasn't had the time to process the trauma while going through treatment and that it needs to process it now.
4 Don't be scared by these flashbacks and don't worry that there is something wrong with you. There isn't anything wrong with you. This is a perfectly normal reaction to have after going through cancer treatment.
5 Talk and write about what you've been through until the intensity of the memory diminishes.
6 Talk about it a lot and talk to a variety of people: a professional therapist or counsellor; friends and family; and people in a support group.
7 Use the Toolkit at the back of the book to help you write about your trauma.

8 Arrange to visit the hospital to update your brain into understanding that the hospital is a safe place to visit.

9 If you are experiencing such debilitating effects from the traumatic reaction that you can't sleep or function day-to-day, talk to your hospital team about a referral to a specialist (such as a clinical psychologist) as there are effective evidence-based treatments to help with trauma reactions.

Notes

Use this page to write about the traumatic aspects of your diagnosis and treatment

8

The physical reminders of breast cancer

Coping with the physical impact of cancer

'The first year after treatment was really hard for me. I felt that I had aged 20 years thanks to the cancer treatment'.

Amy

We've talked a lot about some of the emotions that you might be going through since you completed your treatment, but we all know that it's not just emotional challenges that you can experience once treatment comes to an end. Given what your body is put through during cancer treatment, it's inevitable that there will be some physical side-effects from the treatment that linger around even once treatment has come to an end. Oh joy – breast cancer really is the gift that keeps on giving.

There are some physical side-effects that last for a few weeks, whilst others may continue for months. And sadly, there are some physical side-effects that can go on for years or even become a permanent fixture in your life, especially if you've undergone some form of surgery.

Getting used to physical side-effects and more permanent physical changes, and adapting to these changes on an emotional level are further reasons why it can be so hard to move forward from cancer. Take Toni-Ann for example, who told me that one of the biggest post-treatment challenges that she has faced, has been the return to work. She explained,

'Fatigue and stress levels have made going back to work challenging. Multi-tasking is difficult these days. I was surprised and I didn't expect the return to work to be so hard: I expected to have a month to recover and then be back as normal'.

So, in this chapter we'll look at some of the common physical issues that you might be facing post-treatment, and how you might be able to cope with them. We'll cover:

- Fatigue
- Chemo brain

- Lymphoedema
- Pain or discomfort
- Scars

Fatigue

Let's start with fatigue. Tiredness resulting from cancer treatment is tiredness on a whole other level to regular, every day tiredness. It's like moving through the day whilst up to your waist in thick treacle or mud. And boy, can it be debilitating. It can impact day-to-day life to the point that you're unable to live life in the way that you were before you had cancer. Even doing the simplest of tasks can take it out of you completely: emptying the dishwasher, having a shower, even walking from one room to the next or going up the stairs. Take Kate, for example, who explained:

> 'The thing I found really hard after radiotherapy was the fatigue. For months I suffered with intense fatigue – it was always with me. It took a long time to get my energy levels back to what they'd been before I had cancer'.

For anyone suffering from fatigue after the end of treatment, it can be incredibly frustrating. You've finished treatment and you want to get back to some sort of normality but you're held back by this all-out fatigue. It's preventing you from going back to work, running a household, socializing with your friends, exercising and essentially doing most of the normal day to day things you're longing to do. Your mind wants to move on from cancer and get back to a normal life – but your body can't keep up. For example, Jo L, who was a competitive athlete before she had cancer, explained to me:

> 'Before cancer I played roller derby and competed with my team all over the world. I trained three times a week with the team, I went to the gym three times a week and I walked my dog twice a day. I was living an athletic lifestyle – it was who I was. But since treatment, I'm dealing with fatigue from the medication and my strength and fitness has significantly reduced. I no longer feel like the athlete I once was and I don't know if I'll ever be that person again. I'm trying to deal with this change in my identity'.

How long someone suffers from this fatigue differs from person to person, depending on various factors, including the treatment type and length of treatment they underwent. For many cancer patients, the fatigue can linger around for a while after the end of treatment but it is usual for the fatigue to subside over time.

There's a lot of advice available for someone living with cancer-related fatigue. In fact, one of the major cancer charities has an 83-page booklet on coping with fatigue! But to save you having to read 83 pages about fatigue, here are some tips that I've found from researching around this topic:

- Talk to your cancer medical team or your doctor about your own situation and to eliminate any other underlying causes such as anaemia or thyroid problems.

- Do some exercise. This might sound counter-intuitive, I mean the last thing you feel like doing when you're tired is something known to make you more tired. But actually, there is a lot of research showing that exercise can help with fatigue. Make sure you exercise within your limitations so if you haven't exercised for a while take it easy to start with and gradually build it up. Walking outdoors is a particularly good example of exercise to help with fatigue because not only are you exercising but you are also getting a good dose of fresh air. There are lots of cancer-rehab exercise instructors who help people in your position so it might be worth seeing if there is someone near you who can help you (check their credentials first to make sure they are properly trained in helping people who've had cancer).

- Get enough good quality sleep. This might sound impossible when you're trying to cope with hot flushes and middle-of-the-night-worries, but there are things you can do to help get a good night's sleep. For tips on getting a good night's sleep take a look at the Toolkit at the back of the book.

- Have a healthy diet. If you're not sure where to start with making changes to your diet, talk to your doctor or take advice from a registered dietician. (It's best to get advice from a qualified dietician because there is so much conflicting advice online which can get really confusing).

- Practise self-care. It's easy to put yourself at the bottom of the priority list after your partner, children, job and the dog. Try putting yourself at the top of the list. Recognize your limitations; don't be afraid to say no to things; have a nap if you need it and practise relaxation

- Whilst you're experiencing fatigue, don't expect too much of yourself. Remember to be patient and kind to yourself.

Chemo brain

Chemo brain is a term given to the brain fog that cancer patients can experience due to the impact of certain cancer treatments on brain functionality. Whether brain fog is down to the effect of the chemotherapy drugs on the brain, or a combination of that, plus tiredness, stress, hormonal fluctuations and other chemical changes occurring in the body as a result of treatment, it doesn't matter for the purposes of this section. What matters is that the brain fog which is experienced during treatment, can linger around for a while after the end of treatment. And it's really annoying!

Like fatigue, the frustration associated with living with brain fog can be immense. You've finished treatment and you want to feel normal again. You don't want to go into a room and forget why you went there. You don't want to forget an entire conversation that you had with your mother yesterday. You don't want to misplace your phone yet again (not being able to find your phone while it's in your hand is particularly annoying). You want your brain to function at normal capacity again so that life can feel normal again. Mary told me:

> 'Chemo brain has made working difficult. I'm trying to remain professional and detach cancer from my work, but sometimes I just have to accept that I am not functioning at 100 per cent'.

And Sara explained her chemo brain to me as:

> 'I often have difficulty remembering simple words, the other day I couldn't remember the word for windowsill. I would say this is an everyday occurrence. Sometimes at work I can't think of the word I want to use – only a split second but feels longer. I get really frustrated by it – I want to be me again and be normal again'.

Again, like fatigue, chemo brain can ease over time. However, for those women who go on to take hormone therapy, a side-effect of hormone therapy can be brain fog. So, very annoyingly, it's possible for someone to continue to experience a form of brain fog – whether down to chemotherapy or hormone therapy – for some time. What joy. However, there is advice on coping with brain-fog which includes:

- Make sure you're getting enough rest and good quality sleep (the Toolkit at the back of the book has some advice for a healthy sleep routine).

- Use your brain and exercise your brain by doing puzzles, crosswords and brain games.
- Keep a diary/notebook in which you write down everything that you need to remember. You can record to-do lists, shopping lists, track medication, note upcoming dates and appointments, and generally keep a note of anything you need to remember.
- Your phone can come in really handy here – use the 'notes' App to write notes of what you need to remember, set calendar reminders and alarms.
- Exercise is known to make you feel more alert and decrease tiredness, which will help the chemo brain.
- Don't try to multi-task as this is where things can go horribly wrong. Just focus on the task in hand then move onto the next one.
- Recognize your limitations and don't expect too much of yourself at the moment. Chemo brain does usually improve, just be patient with yourself.
- Talk to your doctor or medical team if you are concerned.

Lymphoedema

Lymphoedema is sadly not unusual in women who've had breast cancer surgery and yet, until you go through breast cancer you may not even have heard of lymphoedema or even the lymphatic system. For those of you who don't know much about it, it's time for a quick biology lesson from Natalie Kruger. Natalie is a Cancer, Palliative Care and Lymphoedema Physiotherapist which basically means she knows an awful lot about lymphoedema.

Natalie explains that the lymphatic system is part of both the circulatory and immune systems in the human body. It has a number of important functions, one of those being to transport lymph fluid throughout the body, draining excess fluid from around your cells, and eventually returning it back to your bloodstream. It does this through small tubes, called lymphatic channels.

Another function of the lymphatic system is something called 'immune surveillance'. Lymph fluid, lymph nodes and lymphatic vessels contain a special type of white blood cell, which are very important for protecting the body against infection.

If the lymphatic system is damaged during cancer treatment, you may be at risk of developing lymphoedema. Lymphoedema is a word used to describe the build-up of lymph fluid under the skin. If lymph nodes have been removed or damaged, often by surgery and/or radiotherapy, you are at risk of developing swelling in that area of the body. For example, if lymph nodes have been removed from your armpit as part of surgery, you are at risk of developing swelling in the breast, chest wall, arm and hand on that side.

There are other risk factors for developing lymphoedema too, such as infection, chemotherapy, not moving or exercising very much or having a higher body mass index. Take Rachel L, for example, who told me about how she came to develop lymphoedema:

'A year ago, I was diagnosed with lymphoedema, triggered by a bout of cellulitis from a very small scratch on my arm. I now have to wear a compression garment. When I first put on the garment, I was really tearful as it hurt my arm and I just couldn't face having to wear it every day for the rest of my life. It reiterated how I was never going to be the same again post-cancer'.

According to Natalie, lymphoedema usually occurs gradually, often within the first year or two of treatment, though the risk is generally considered to be life-long. And although the swelling may come and go at first, if it's not treated early, it can become more severe and persistent. She says that while there is no cure for lymphoedema, it can be well managed with skin care (to prevent infection), compression garments, exercise, maintaining a healthy body weight and manual or self-lymphatic drainage (a special type of massage). Surgery may also be an option, although it is not routinely available on the NHS.

The important thing is, if you are at risk of developing lymphoedema, or are showing early signs of swelling, contact your local lymphoedema service early. The earlier the swelling is treated, the easier it will be to take care of in the future. Ask your doctor for a referral to your local NHS lymphoedema clinic or private lymphoedema practitioner. If you're not sure whether a service or clinic exists in your area, check out an online directory – the Useful Resources section at the back of the book includes some suggestions.

If you develop lymphoedema, not only can it be uncomfortable and sometimes painful, but it can also make you feel unattractive and self-conscious. It can also, sadly, be another reminder of what cancer has done to you. When I talked to Molly about her lymphoedema, she explained:

'One of the biggest post-treatment challenges for me has been coping with lymphoedema in my hand and arm. It's a huge problem for me as it brings up several issues: it's a constant reminder of cancer, I feel betrayed by my body and I'm very self-conscious about it'.

Whilst it's important to get expert advice and treatment for lymphoedema, Natalie's top tips for managing lymphoedema at home are:

- Look after your skin to reduce the risk of infection.
- Exercise to keep the lymph moving around the body.
- Maintain a healthy body weight.
- Elevate the swollen area when possible.
- Wear compression daily, or as directed by your lymphoedema practitioner.

The Useful Resources section at the back of this book contains plenty of resources to support you in learning more about lymphoedema.

Pain or discomfort

If you've had surgery, chemotherapy or radiotherapy then there's a good chance that you might still feel pain or discomfort when you reach the end of your treatment. For example, scar tissue and long-term seromas can be painful; radiotherapy can cause blisters; chemotherapy can cause peripheral neuropathy which is the pain, numbness and tingling in hands, arms and feet; and reconstruction sites can be numb and uncomfortable. While talking to Lindsey about the lingering side-effects, she said:

'My biggest challenge post treatment has been the ongoing issues with my reconstruction which has caused me daily pain'.

It's not only the lingering side-effects from completed treatment that can cause you pain or discomfort, some of the longer-term medication can cause joint aches and bone pain. Regardless of the cause, the intensity of pain and discomfort varies from person to person. But whatever the intensity, it's another reminder of cancer and something else that might hinder you from moving on fully. One of the women I talked to in writing this book commented:

'I had a double mastectomy and reconstruction, but I'm still trying to get used to my new breasts: I don't feel like they are part of me. My entire chest is completely numb and it doesn't feel like it's part of my body. Aesthetically I may look the same as I did before I had cancer, but I feel entirely different'.

Continuing to experience pain and discomfort even after the end of treatment can be really disheartening: you've completed your treatment and you just want to move on from cancer, but thanks to how your body is physically feeling, you're reminded of it on a daily basis.

In many instances, these issues can resolve themselves but it is important that if you are suffering from pain or discomfort that you speak to your doctor or medical team.

Scars[1]

Some scars are big, some are small. Some scars are on a part of the body for all the world to see, others are for your eyes only. Regardless of their size and location, scars can be problematic in a number of ways.

Firstly, there is the sensation of the scar and its surrounding area. The area around a scar can be numb and feel disconnected. On the other hand, it's not uncommon to feel tightness, discomfort and pain in the scar area which can persist for years after an operation.

Secondly, it's not unusual to experience mobility issues and to feel a pulling sensation in the scar area which is due to something called an adhesion. This is where two internal surfaces that are not usually connected, stick to each other.

Thirdly, internal scar tissue can extend beyond the surgical site and thus problems from scars can extend beyond the scar area itself. For example, scarring can interrupt the lymphatic pathways and cause lymphoedema. And where healthy parts of the body are having to work harder to make up for the lack of movement in the scar area, this can cause irritation and fatigue.

However your scars feel, whatever the impact of them on your body and whatever they represent to you, scars from cancer treatment are things that will be with you forever. But, the period immediately after the end of treatment can be a period of adjustment to these scars and their impact upon you. If you're struggling with your scars, here are a few tips:

- If your scar, or the surrounding area, is painful or uncomfortable then you should speak to your doctor or medical team.
- Scar tissue massage therapy might be an option if you are experiencing numbness, pain, tightness or pulling in the area of your scar. This essentially involves a qualified therapist using special, gentle massage techniques to bring nutrients into the scar area and encourage blood and lymphatic flow which can initiate further healing by gently working to encourage the scar tissue to become loose and mobile. It can also improve the way the scar looks. Ask your doctor or medical team about this.
- If you are upset by the presence of your scars, you could consider talking to a counsellor or therapist.
- Try to reframe the idea that scars are a sign of cancer, into them being a symbol of rejuvenation and recovery: Scars show how amazing our bodies are at overcoming the worst and bouncing back.

All in all, there are plenty of lingering physical side-effects from cancer treatment. You may be experiencing other side-effects not covered in this chapter. Whatever you're facing, the key is to seek professional help if these physical side-effects become problematic.

Top tip
Be patient with yourself and your physical recovery.

Checklist

Here's a recap of the key points for you to take away from this chapter.

1 Speak to your medical team or doctor about any lingering physical pain or discomfort.
2 When it comes to rebuilding your strength, think of it as a gradual process. Do it slowly with small goals.
3 Practise self-care and make sure that you rest when you need to. Remember the saying, 'You can't pour from an empty cup'.
4 Ensure that you are getting a good night's sleep every night. This can be tricky with some of the physical and mental challenges that you're

facing, but the Toolkit at the back of the book has some helpful tips on getting a good night's sleep.

5 Have a healthy diet. There's a lot of unhelpful nutritional advice for people who've had breast cancer or cancer generally. Stick to the reputable sources of information: seek professional advice, ask your doctor or look at the list of resources in the Useful Resources at the back of the book.

6 There is support available for most – if not all – the physical issues that you might be dealing with. Ask your hospital team or your doctor for referrals, recommendations and advice.

Notes

Use this page for your notes on coping with the physical impact of cancer

9

Changes to your physical appearance

Coping with changes to your physical appearance

'Going through hair regrowth, having the tell-tale puffy steroid face, having no eyebrows or eyelashes and wearing a compression garment for lymphoedema in my hand and arm is all hard for me. The changes in my physical appearance since the end of treatment have been a massive identity adjustment that people just don't seem to understand. I keep waiting for the day when I will recognize myself in the mirror again'.

Molly

Treatment may be over, but you might still be exhibiting some changes to your physical appearance in addition to scarring that we looked at in the previous chapter. For example, you may have lost your hair through chemotherapy and now it's only just starting to grow back, if at all or in a different colour/style to your old one. Molly experienced this, and she told me:

'I did the cold cap through chemotherapy and thankfully kept a lot of my hair, but it thinned and it now looks weird because it's grey and it's partly long, partly growing back. Every time I look in the mirror, I do a double take because I don't look like me'.

You may have blistering from radiotherapy or changes to your body shape as a result of surgery. You may have lost your eyebrows and eyelashes during chemotherapy and they have yet to grow back. And you might have gained or lost weight during treatment. The weight gain from breast cancer treatment (and then from the use of certain post-treatment hormone therapies) is one of the most common pain points that I came across in my interviews with the women for this book. For example, Cathy told me:

'I have body confidence issues since finishing my cancer treatment, especially around weight gain. I'm the heaviest I've ever been and I can't seem to turn it around'.

And Sara explained:

> 'Another thing that cancer has changed, is the weight gain that I just can't shift despite being incredibly active and eating a really healthy diet'.

Whatever the changes, if you don't look like yourself, how can you feel like yourself? And if you look different to the pre-cancer version of yourself, you might find that people continue to treat you differently when all you want is to be treated the way in which you were treated before you had cancer. Changes in your physical appearance can be yet another hindrance to moving beyond cancer.

Worrying about your appearance is perfectly natural. It's not vain, it's normal. It's especially natural for women to worry about their appearance when it affects parts of the body associated with their femininity such as a reconstructed breast, wearing a prosthetic breast or being flat chested; a bald head or wearing a wig; a lack of eyebrows and eyelashes; a change in weight or wearing a compression garment.

Furthermore, changes to your appearance can cause a myriad of emotions. You can feel loss at losing part of your body, for example a breast, due to a mastectomy. You can feel disgust at the scars left behind after surgery. You can feel sad that you're no longer the same person looking back from the mirror. You can feel embarrassed about people seeing or noticing the changes in your appearance. You can find it difficult to adapt to the new version of your appearance.

When I spoke to Nevo who had breast cancer 10 years ago and who is, incidentally, an image consultant/stylist and body confidence coach who helps women post breast cancer treatment she told me,

> 'I attended a couple of post-breast cancer courses when I finished my treatment and I was surprised that they didn't include a talk or session on body confidence. Specialists came to the courses to talk to us about diet and exercise but there was no mention of how to regain your confidence. They didn't talk about restyling after surgery, how to dress after a mastectomy or lumpectomy, weight gain or loss due to treatment, how to look at your body in the mirror, how to cope with the feeling of dissociation from your body, how to reclaim and reconnect with your body and how to look at your body positively. As a body confidence coach myself, I see this part of the recovery process as being incredibly important'.

To help in coping with these changes, Dr Jane Clark is back again to provide some advice on coping with these emotions.

Loss and guilt

According to Jane, you often hear people say things like, 'I'm grateful they took my breast because that saved my life, and at least I'm still here'. What they don't say is how distraught they are over the loss of their breast or how they hate looking at their body in a mirror, having their partner see them naked or trying to find clothing that camouflages the asymmetry in their chest area. Many people feel guilty for complaining about the way their looks have changed, because they think that they should be thankful that they're still alive.

But it's okay to be sad about the way your appearance has changed and it's important to acknowledge the loss of the way you used to look so that you can grieve for this loss. It could be the loss of one or both breasts, it could be the loss of your hair, eyebrows and eyelashes, or it could be the weight gain or loss from the treatment. Regardless of the way in which your appearance has changed, the important thing is to acknowledge that you have lost part of your appearance and you can then grieve for it. Grief can involve so many emotions and allowing yourself to move through these emotions with compassion, kindness and support can help. Shed the tears that need to be shed and nurture yourself through this process.

Difficulty accepting the change

Sometimes people find it really hard to accept a change to their physical appearance whether that's different hair growing back after chemo or a change in their body shape due to surgery. They may even feel disgust and revulsion at the changes. Jane says that these are perfectly normal reactions – especially if the change is a major change to their body shape. After all, they probably looked the same for many years before this change.

In this situation, Jane's advice is to try to think about body acceptance on a sliding continuum from 'absolute detest' all the way to 'loving your body'. You might be at the 'absolute detest' end of the scale and you're not going to reach the 'loving your body' end of the scale in a day (or even ever). It's a gradual process of moving along the spectrum and there may be days when you feel less far along the spectrum and days when you feel more tolerant of your changed body. You just need to start off by trying to move the sliding scale from absolute detest to, perhaps being able to tolerate your new appearance. Be kind to yourself. Work on this in small increments and don't put yourself under pressure.

Inability to look at surgical scars

Some people cannot look at their scars or touch them. They are horrified by them. Don't worry, Jane says that this is a perfectly normal reaction. Her advice is to start by acknowledging this reaction. Then you can move onto something called 'graded exposure'. Let's use the example of a mastectomy scar. Start by looking at the outline of your chest while it's covered up. Try to be curious about the new shape and how it's different to before. Then, when you are comfortable doing this, expose one end of the scar and look at that. Look at it in the mirror and without a mirror. Touch the scar and get used to how it feels. Be curious about the scar without being judgmental – don't think of it as ugly, just try to describe what is there without judging it or labelling it as 'unattractive' (or giving it any other label). Then do the same with the other end of the scar.

Gradually expose more of the scar using this process, until you've uncovered the whole scar and you can look at it in its entirety. By doing this, you are gradually desensitizing your brain to the change and you won't feel as overwhelmed by it. You can do this over a period of days or weeks, or you can do it all in one day. It's important to go at your own pace and do what's right for you.

Loss of identity, self or femininity

Jane notes that changes to your physical appearance might cause you to feel damaged or that you've lost an important part of your identity, self or even femininity. But remember that your appearance is only one part of you and you are made up from so many other parts. You're focusing on the one part of you that's changed and you're forgetting everything else – the other parts of your body, your mind, your personality, your character, who you are and what you stand for as a person.

Jane's advice is to, instead, imagine you're in a dark room and there is a spotlight shining on the part of your body that you are struggling to accept. Now expand the spotlight so that it includes another part of you. Remind yourself that there are other parts of you. Then do it again and again and again. Each time, focus on another part of your body, your mind or you as a person. The part that you don't like is only one small part of you and there is so much more.

Dressing to feel your best

Just a quick note here to remind you that the way you dress can help with body confidence. For example, wearing clothes that fit your new body shape will give you a confidence boost. Maybe try consulting a personal stylist (clothes shops often offer this service free of charge) or take a good friend whose opinion you value. If your hair isn't growing back, or it's growing back slowly, you can try different options – scarves, wigs, hats – to work out what feels right for you at this stage. It's all your own personal choice and up to you what feels right.

Coping with reconstruction

It's not unusual for it to take a little while to get used to new sensations if you've had reconstructive surgery. Taking a reconstructed breast as an example, Jane advises that it will take time for the brain to assimilate and make sense of the reconstructed breast. So, you might start off with a reconstructed breast feeling like, for example, a small beanbag is sitting on your chest. Try to acknowledge this feeling without fear or judgment. In other words, try not to label it as weird, disgusting or unpleasant, but just notice that your reconstructed breast feels this particular way today. As you notice these sensations over a period of time, you will notice that your brain will gradually adapt to your reconstructed breast and it will no longer feel like a separate part of you. The key here is to allow your brain the time to adapt.

Top tip

No matter how the changes in your physical appearance affect you, remember to be patient with your body: acknowledge the loss or change and remember that you'll find your way through this.

Checklist

Here's a recap of the key points for you to take away from this chapter.

1 Don't put yourself under any pressure when it comes to dealing with changes to your physical appearance

2 In relation to the more permanent changes to your physical appearance it's okay to feel sadness and grief.

3 You can work on coming to terms with permanent changes slowly – there is no need to rush.

4 Talk to your friends and family about how you feel so that they understand and can be sensitive to your feelings.

5 Be patient with your body: acknowledge the loss or change and remember that you'll find your way through it.

Notes

Use this page for your notes on coping with changes to your physical appearance

10

The menopause and hormone therapy

Understanding the impact of hormone therapy and coping with the side-effects

'When I was diagnosed with breast cancer I had absolutely no expectation that going through treatment would kick-start the menopause for me. It didn't cross my mind. The menopause is something that old women go through silently, stoically and without making a fuss. I'm 43 years old, which is certainly not the typical menopausal age'.

Taken from Ticking Off Breast Cancer

Before being diagnosed with breast cancer you probably had no idea that a major impact of breast cancer treatment could be an early menopause. And not only is it early – by which I mean you go through the menopause before your body would naturally go through it – but the symptoms can be particularly intense. Breast cancer really is the gift that just keeps giving, isn't it?

You might be experiencing menopausal symptoms and want to know what you can do to cope with these, but before we look at some coping tips, it's interesting to know what's actually happening in your body. So, I've enlisted the help of Dr Sophie McGrath again (she's the Consultant Medical Oncologist at the Royal Marsden NHS Foundation Trust who's helped out in some of the previous chapters) to help explain everything.[1] There's quite a bit to cover, so we're going to divide it into these five manageable sections:

- What exactly is the menopause?
- How surgery and chemotherapy can cause a temporary menopause.
- Hormone therapy: the different types of hormone therapy and how hormone therapy can induce a temporary menopause or mimic menopausal symptoms.
- Common side-effects of hormone therapy.
- Tips for alleviating the common side-effects.

What exactly is the menopause?

As Sophie explains, simply put, when a woman gets to around the age of fifty,[2] her ovaries naturally stop producing as much of the hormone oestrogen. As you probably know, this means that the ovaries stop releasing eggs and so a woman's periods stop. But there is more to the menopause than no more periods. Oestrogen plays a role in many of the body's functions, for example in the regulation of the body's internal temperature thermostat. So, when oestrogen is in decline, it's natural to experience some changes within your body. These are often called menopausal symptoms and they include things like hot flushes, aching joints, fatigue and weight gain.

How surgery and chemotherapy can cause a temporary menopause

Some surgeries and chemotherapy drugs can induce the menopause in women by causing the ovaries to stop producing oestrogen – there are various ways in which this can happen but we don't need to go into those here. The point is, that because the menopause is prematurely imposed by treatment, its symptoms can be more intense, with a faster onset than a natural menopause. So, you might come out of breast cancer treatment in an induced menopause and suffering from some of the symptoms mentioned later in this chapter.

Sophie explains that if you're not taking hormone therapy (because you don't have oestrogen positive breast cancer) this surgical/chemotherapy menopause may be temporary: you may start your periods again, and all symptoms will cease. In some women, periods return a couple of months after chemotherapy whilst in others it can be up to two years after chemotherapy, depending on age. For example, younger women may have a return of periods sooner, whilst periods may cease permanently for women approaching menopause around the age of 51 (51 is the average age for a woman to start the menopause).

However, if, when you finish your active treatment, you are put onto certain hormone therapies, this may extend the temporary menopause caused by surgery or chemotherapy, because, according to Sophie, certain hormone therapies can mimic the menopause.

Hormone therapy

Let's talk a little bit about hormone therapy here because interestingly, there is not just a one-size-fits-all hormone therapy, but rather a few varied types which do different things within the body. I don't know about you, but it confused me as to why I was on a particular hormone therapy whilst someone else of a similar age, was on something different. So, I asked Sophie to explain…

'Oestrogen is present in everyone to differing extents. In women who haven't been through the menopause – pre-menopausal women – oestrogen is mainly produced in the ovaries. In women who've been through the menopause – post-menopausal women – and in men, some oestrogen is made within the body fat. The hormone oestrogen is known to stimulate the growth of some – not all – breast cancer cells. All breast cancer patients are tested to see whether their breast cancer is the type of breast cancer that is stimulated to grow by oestrogen, that is to say whether they have 'oestrogen positive' breast cancer.

Hormone therapy is usually only given to patients who have oestrogen positive breast cancer – whether they are pre-menopausal, post-menopausal or diagnosed whilst going through the menopause.

There are a number of different types of hormone therapy and they each work differently. Firstly, hormone therapy can reduce or stop the production of oestrogen within the body: Zoladex[3] reduces brain (pituitary) stimulation to the ovaries so they stop producing oestrogen whereas the Aromatase Inhibitors – Anastrozole, Letrozole and Exemestane – stop the production of oestrogen from testosterone within body fat. Secondly, hormone therapy can work by blocking the oestrogen from entering into cancer cells and stimulating their growth (for example, Tamoxifen).

The type of hormone therapy given to a breast cancer patient depends on many factors. It depends upon particular factors within the cancer, the age of the patient, whether the patient is pre- or post-menopausal, the patient's risk of recurrence, the patient's personal health history and the preferences of the oncologist and their institution. Oncologists sometimes use tools such as Nottingham Prognostic Index and NHS-Predict[4] or more detailed molecular tests to help calculate an individual patient's risk of future breast cancer recurrence, and the potential prognostic benefit of taking hormone therapy.

Hormone therapy is given for a number of years – usually five to ten years – to help prevent the cancer returning. Some hormone therapy drugs are taken as a daily tablet and some are administered as a regular injection. Hormone therapies can be given singularly – only one type of therapy – or may be prescribed as a combination of two therapies. It's also possible that during the course of the five to ten years, someone will change from one type of hormone therapy to another. This could be down to a variety of factors, including whether the woman is considered to have gone through the menopause during the course of treatment, her overall health situation, or her tolerance of the medication's side-effects.

Approximately 70 per cent of breast cancer cases are oestrogen positive, so there is a high proportion of people who are on hormone therapy after breast cancer treatment'.

Side-effects

If you're taking hormone therapy for breast cancer, the chances are that you will experience some side-effects – not everyone does, but side-effects are common. The side-effects of breast cancer hormone therapy are very similar to menopausal symptoms because, as Sophie explains, essentially the hormone therapy is either pushing your body into a form of medically-induced menopause (by stopping the body from producing oestrogen) or mimicking many of the symptoms experienced in menopause, due to reduced oestrogen impact on the cells of the body.

Furthermore, Sophie says that it's possible that you will experience these side-effects for as long as you are taking the hormone therapy. So, if you start taking hormone therapy at the age of 30, for 10 years, you could experience menopausal-type side-effects for the 10 years that you are on the hormone therapy. You may then come off hormone therapy only to find yourself going through a natural menopause some years later.

According to Sophie, if you're pre-menopausal when you start hormone therapy, it's possible to go through 'the menopause' whilst taking the hormone therapy so that when you finish your hormone therapy, you will come out as post-menopausal. You will have been through the menopause but not know it because the menopausal symptoms that you're experiencing for the entire period that you've been on hormone therapy will have masked any symptoms associated with a natural menopause. Thus, women on hormone therapy over the average menopausal age (between 45 and 55 years old) may sometimes (depending upon the hormone therapy they are on) have blood tests to check their menopausal status. If these blood tests confirm that the woman has become post-menopausal whilst on hormone therapy, then she may have her hormone therapy changed. For example, most pre-menopausal women have Tamoxifen and if they become post-menopausal whilst taking Tamoxifen, they may be changed to an Aromatase Inhibitor.

Sophie explains that if you've already been through a natural menopause when you have breast cancer treatment – i.e., you're post-menopausal – you will still be prescribed hormone therapy if your breast cancer is oestrogen positive. This is because although the ovaries are no longer producing oestrogen, oestrogen can still be produced in the body from other hormones such as testosterone in body fat. Going on hormone treatment as a post-menopausal woman can still cause some menopausal symptoms. Rachel L had already been through a natural menopause before having breast cancer, and she told me:

'I went through early menopause at the age of thirty-nine before I had cancer, so I was put on Letrozole which is the hormone treatment for post-menopausal women. The side-effects from being on Letrozole are far more intense than the symptoms I experienced when going through the menopause. The hot flushes are hotter and the aches and pains in my joints are more painful'.

Common side-effects[5] of hormone therapy and the menopause

Different hormone therapies can have different side-effects and, as with everything in the cancer world, people react differently to hormone therapies. So, while someone might have little or no side-effects, someone else on the same therapy could be experiencing a range of unpleasant ones. Side-effects vary from person to person, and not everyone will experience them all. Some of the common side-effects are:

- Hot flushes during the day
- Night sweats
- Experiencing an emotional rollercoaster
- Brain fog
- Decreased concentration and attention span
- Short term memory loss
- Disturbed sleep and insomnia
- Painful joints
- Erratic periods or periods stopping entirely
- Fatigue and tiredness

- Weight gain
- Decreased sex drive
- Vaginal dryness
- Increased anxiety
- Bone thinning leading to osteopenia and osteoporosis

As you can see, hormone therapy and the menopause can bring some pretty unpleasant things to the party and these side-effects can be a real struggle for some. Let's take a closer look at some of these side-effects (remembering that people will have different experiences).

First up are our dear friends, the hot flushes (or hot flashes as they are also called). These vary in intensity and frequency from person to person. They range from a little flush of heat which can be dissipated by the mere wave of a fan, all the way up to cruel, intense, burning flashes rising up from the feet to the tip of the scalp involving lots of sweat. They can hit completely out of the blue at any point during the day, with no regard to what you might be doing. Mary was 27 when she starting taking Tamoxifen and she told me:

'I've been experiencing a few menopausal symptoms such as hot flushes, night sweats, body aches and being tired! My hot flushes have been intense'.

Night sweats are essentially hot flushes that occur at night but they can feel more intense in the middle of the night compared to those that occur during the day. They can drench you, your night clothes and bedding in sweat. Kate told me that she'd been experiencing night sweats, she said:

'Since starting Tamoxifen I've experienced really fierce hot flushes, especially at night. Sometimes I wake up in the night and everything is just drenched in sweat and the heat coming off my body is intense'.

When these night sweats happen every night, there's no chance of having a full night of sleep which just adds to the general feeling of 'bleurgh' because now you're having to cope with tiredness on top of everything else. Oh, and by the way, insomnia itself is also a side-effect. Great.

Next up is the emotional rollercoaster. Your emotions can turn upside-down, back-to-front and inside-out. Life can become an emotional rollercoaster with unfamiliar highs and lows. One minute you can be laughing out loud at something someone has sent to you on your phone, and the next minute you're crying because an advert for a donkey sanctuary has come on the television. As with everything, the intensity of emotions will differ from person to person.

Another side-effect is anxiety. If it's not bad enough to have increased anxiety as a result of having had cancer, it's also possible to experience increased levels of anxiety as a result of taking hormone therapy. The levels of anxiety range from that just bubbling under the surface, up to crippling levels. But because anxiety is such a common lingering side-effect of cancer treatment generally, who knows whether your anxiety is down to having had cancer or as a direct result of the hormone therapy. What joy.

Vaginal dryness causing pain and discomfort during intercourse, and a loss of libido are common side-effects and yes that can mean drying up down there and never ever wanting to have sex ever again. Inevitably this can then lead to feelings of low self-worth, frustration, resentment, inadequacy, together with relationship issues. Take this comment received from one of the women I interviewed:

> I've been on Letrozole for three years and one of the most significant side-effects for me has been the vaginal dryness and lack of sex drive. Sexual intercourse is really painful for me now and this has led to marital tensions'.

And this is certainly not the only comment that someone made along these lines.

And then there are the memory issues – in addition to a decrease in concentration and your attention span, it can feel like a fog has descended on your brain making you forget names, where you left the pile of clean washing and other short term memory loss. Rachel L told me:

> 'I'm really forgetful. I have terrible brain fog and I can no longer multi-task. I've had to change the way I work as I know I can't do two things at the same time'.

Joint pain can be minimal or severe – so severe that it can sometimes have a debilitating impact on day-to-day activities. A loss in bone density increases the risk of osteopenia and osteoporosis. Oh, and let's not forget that hormone therapy can cause weight gain. Cathy told me that she was finding the weight gain to be particularly problematic. She explained:

> I have body confidence issues since finishing my cancer treatment, especially around weight gain. I'm the heaviest I've ever been and I can't seem to turn it around'.

And just to make it harder to deal with all the other side-effects, the menopause and hormone therapy can drain you of all energy, making you permanently tired and fatigued where it regularly feels like you're walking through treacle just to get to the end of the day. Take Jo L, for example, who described her experience on Tamoxifen to me:

'Tamoxifen is having a massive impact on me. It's made me feel light headed, dizzy and fatigued. It makes me feel like a different person physically'.

Not only are all these side-effects distressing, unpleasant and annoying, but being induced into a menopause before you reach the time in life to go through it naturally, can be incredibly upsetting. Aside from the obvious fertility issues, for some women it represents a major turning point in life from being young(ish) and feeling like you still have plenty of time ahead of you to becoming, well, past-it. In fact, tragically, many women report that they experience so many intense side-effects that they forget who they really are and 'lose' the real them.

Hormone Replacement Therapy (HRT)

For women who go through a natural menopause and haven't had a hormone-related cancer, hormone replacement therapy (also known as HRT) is often prescribed for them to help counter the menopausal symptoms. In simple terms, HRT essentially replaces the oestrogen that the body is no longer making, allowing all those internal body functions that require oestrogen, to continue to function as if the body hadn't stopped making its own oestrogen. This can go a long way in countering many of the menopausal symptoms.

Generally speaking, according to Sophie, it's not advised for a woman who has had oestrogen positive breast cancer to take HRT because the whole point of hormone therapy is either to stop the production of oestrogen or block its effect on cells. This means that there isn't an obvious choice of treatment to help women who are experiencing menopausal symptoms as a result of being on hormone therapy. It can, therefore, mean that women on hormone therapy struggle with many of the side-effects.

Tips for alleviating the common side-effects

Unfortunately, there isn't a magic pill or a quick fix when it comes to the side-effects of hormone therapy. And sadly, there isn't a whole lot of support freely or readily available for women experiencing these side-effects as a result of hormone therapy. As a result, lots of women tend to take the view that they're so grateful to be alive after having had cancer and so grateful to the hormone therapy for helping to minimize the risk of recurrence, that they will put up with the side-effects. I spoke to Amy and Cathy about this, and Amy told me:

> 'Unfortunately, hormone therapy is all part of the breast cancer package for me and if it's helping to prevent my cancer from returning then I'll learn to cope with whatever side-effects get thrown my way'.

Whilst Cathy said:

> 'Before cancer I'd always worked and in fact, I was ambitious and had a strong work ethic. However, I found it really hard to get back to work due to the side-effects of the Aromatase Inhibitors that I was on. I suffered from hot flushes, aches and pains and intense tiredness. But I can live my life with the security that they're helping to stop the cancer coming back. This has helped me cope with taking them'.

But it doesn't have to be this way. There are natural ways to counter some of the side-effects, there are lifestyle changes that can help and, at the end of the day, it's really important to seek professional help if your quality of life is suffering badly as a result of the side-effects of your hormone therapy. As a starting point, Sophie and I have put together the following tips to help you, but we urge you to speak to your medical team if you're struggling. There is no reason for you to suffer in silence.

Hot flushes and night sweats

Hot flushes during the day and night sweats can be triggered by certain things such as caffeine, alcohol and spicy foods. Try to work out what your triggers are, so that you can cut down these things. For night sweats, you can keep a small can of water spray next to your bed, have a fan in the bedroom and use a specially designed cooling pillow. Bamboo nightwear can also help because it is highly breathable, absorbent and temperature-regulating. If you are sweating and having to change clothes in the middle of the night, then wearing this might help. Speak to your oncology team as they may be able to suggest other ways of helping with hot flushes and night sweats, such as acupuncture – which has really helped me – and medication.

Bone density

For those of you who may not be familiar with this term, let me explain what is meant by bone density. In simple terms, bones are living, growing tissue made from protein and minerals. Higher bone mineral content means denser bones. And the denser your bones, the stronger they generally are, meaning that they are less likely to break. Aromatase Inhibitor hormone therapy, as well as the menopause, can reduce your bone density over time making your bones weaker and more susceptible to breakage. That is to say, the use of Aromatase Inhibitors – and likewise the menopause itself – can lead to a condition called osteoporosis and its precursor, osteopenia. To help prevent the onset of osteopenia or osteoporosis, the advice is to:

- Ensure you have enough vitamin D and calcium in your diet – check with your doctor or oncologist about whether supplements are suitable for you and you may wish to consider taking advice from a specialist registered dietician or nutritionist about which supplements would help.
- Do gentle weight bearing exercises – again check with a professional if you have had recent surgery, are now at risk of lymphoedema, or having treatment.
- Stop smoking.
- Avoid excess alcohol.
- Keep to a healthy weight.

It's also worth talking to your oncology team about having Dexa scans to monitor your bone strength. A Dexa – or bone density – scan is a quick and painless procedure that involves lying on your back on an X-ray table so an area of your body can be scanned. It compares your bone density with the bone density expected for a healthy adult of your own age, gender and ethnicity. The results indicate whether you have the bone density expected of someone of your age, gender and ethnicity and they can also identify whether you are within the parameters of osteopenia or osteoporosis. If the scan shows that your bone density is lower than it should be, additional bone strengthening medication may be necessary.

Brain fog

It's common to experience brain fog as a result of the menopause or hormone therapy. This brain fog can be confused with lingering chemo brain if you've only recently completed chemotherapy. They both cause the same fogginess, an inability to recall names or words, and a general inability to use your brain as you used to before cancer. Exercise can help, as can CBT – cognitive behavioural therapy with a trained professional – and mindfulness to reduce stress. It's worth understanding that if you're experiencing brain fog, you might need to adapt how you work and how you live generally. For example, avoid multitasking, make to-do lists, and don't arrange work meetings at times of the day when the brain fog is at its worst. There is an increasing awareness and acknowledgement by the medical profession of this symptom and a number of hospitals and clinics offer courses to help.

Weight gain

This is a particularly prevalent side-effect of Tamoxifen. With less oestrogen entering the cells of your body, your metabolism slows down and you can put on weight more easily – especially around the waist. And it can be really hard to lose this weight. But it is possible by exercising – especially weight bearing exercises – and making healthy changes to your diet. It's advisable to take professional advice from your oncology team or a registered dietician about making changes to your diet.

Aching joints

Aching joints are often worse in the morning but they can improve over the course of the day with increased exercise and movement. To help with aching joints, keep yourself active within your limits: do plenty of exercise but recognize that you may not be able to exercise at the same level as pre-cancer. It's worth consulting your oncology team to ask for advice on supplements and acupuncture.

Vaginal dryness

It is very common to experience vaginal dryness which can lead to painful or uncomfortable sexual intercourse as well as general discomfort. Ask your doctor or oncology team about safe vaginal lubricants and moisturizers to use to help with the vaginal dryness. Talk to your oncology team about this side-effect because early, regular use of vaginal moisturizers and additional lubricants prior to intercourse can really help. Yes, it might feel totally embarrassing to talk to them about it but honestly you won't be alone in asking these questions and this is the sort of information that they can help provide. There are some additional resources included in the Useful Resources section at the back of the book.

Anxiety

For advice on coping with increased anxiety, take a look at the chapter on anxiety (Chapter 4).

Disturbed sleep and insomnia

For advice on getting a better night's sleep look at the sleep section of the Toolkit at the back of the book.

Top tip

Don't suffer in silence: seek help.

Checklist

Here's a recap of the key points for you to take away from this chapter and some further tips for coping with menopausal symptoms generally.

1 The topic of the menopause and hormone therapy is quite complicated and everyone's situation is different. It's important to talk to
   your medical team with any questions or concerns about your own
   situation.
2 Fertility issues associated with taking hormone therapy or as a result
   of an induced menopause are beyond the remit of this book. It is
   important to seek professional advice in relation to fertility – you can
   be referred to a specialist by your oncologist.
3 Talk to your oncologist or doctor about any natural supplements or
   other medication that you could take to reduce the symptoms.
4 Acupuncture, reflexology, CBT (cognitive behavioural therapy) and
   hypnotherapy are all known to help ease menopausal symptoms
   in some women. Ask your doctor or oncologist whether there are

any local services available for women who've had breast cancer – sometimes they are available at local day hospices or cancer support centres.

5   Ensure that you're eating a good healthy balanced diet and exercising regularly and try to avoid sudden extreme diets that your body is not used to.

6   Allow the side-effects of hormone therapy and menopausal symptoms to settle down over time. A lot of women say that the first six months to a year are the worst time for intense side-effects from hormone therapy but that it then gets easier after time. If this isn't the case for you, consult your doctor or oncologist.

7   Some women find that varying brands of Tamoxifen affect them differently so that the side-effects are less intense on one brand of Tamoxifen compared to others. This is all down to each individual. If you want to try different brands then it is worth continuing with each for a couple of months in order to assess the effect. Some – but not all – pharmacists can source different brands and some – but not all – doctors will prescribe specific ones. This is something that you can discuss with your doctor and pharmacist.

8   It's important to be aware of the more serious side-effects of some of the hormone therapy drugs such as the risk of endocrine cancers and blood clots from Tamoxifen. In terms of endocrine cancers there is a direct correlation between length of time on Tamoxifen and the risk of endometrial cancer – the biggest risk is for those on Tamoxifen for over 10 years, so women are rarely kept on it for that long. You should seek urgent doctor/oncologist review if you develop new vaginal bleeding/spotting whilst on Tamoxifen. In terms of blood clots, there is an increased risk of deep vein thrombosis blood clots – especially in the leg, so it's important to educate yourself on the steps to minimize the risk of a blood clot during day-to-day life and for example, traveling by plane.

9   If the side-effects are getting you down or are getting in the way of your daily life, it's important to seek professional advice (whether that is the doctor, oncologist, menopause specialist and/or a counsellor). Your oncologist might give you a short-term break from the treatment to allow the side-effects to settle and then perhaps start you on a different brand of the same treatment or an alternative

hormone treatment. However, it is important to only have a break from the treatment in collaboration with your oncology team.

10 A lot of women correlate the menopause with getting old. Don't allow the menopause or the impact of hormone therapy to represent being old, past-it or beyond your prime. View it as just another step in your life. You're not past your prime. You're just reaching the prime of your life. Hold your head up high, adjust your crown and proudly move forward to make the most of the rest of your life.

Notes

Note down the lifestyle changes you plan to incorporate into daily life to help with your menopausal symptoms.

11

Loneliness

You can have the best, most wonderful, loving friends and family and yet still feel lonely

'After treatment finished, I stayed off work for a while longer. I wasn't busy because I was tired and so I had plenty of free time in which to analyse everything that had happened over the previous few months. I remember one day I just felt so desperate and alone, I didn't know what to do with myself and I just cried all day. And then I cried every day for a week'.

Jo H

From the moment you were diagnosed with cancer, the chances are that you'll have had a network of support from loving family members and fantastic friends. You probably had plenty of help with things such as taking you to hospital, walking the dog, or home-cooked meals delivered to your door step. Caring for, and supporting, a loved one through cancer treatment is where many people really step up and show their worth. Such support and kindness is amazing, wonderful and enormously appreciated. In fact, you can feel like you're wrapped up on a warm, safe, comfort blanket of love and support.

However, as treatment ends, it's not unusual for your friends and family to back off a bit: for them to expect you to be back to normal and to appear less supportive than perhaps they were during the course of your treatment. The telephone calls and checking-in texts can dry up, the visits can tail-off and the offers of help fade away. But sadly, for many people who've just finished cancer treatment, the end of treatment can be a time when support from family and friends is needed more than ever. With less support from friends and family, not only can you feel like you've been set adrift by the hospital, it can also feel that you no longer have the life vest of support from your loved ones around you. This can inevitably lead to feelings of loneliness and thoughts such as:

- My friends have drifted away since treatment ended, even though it's the time when I need them most.
- My friends don't understand what I'm going through.
- My friends expect me to be back to normal but I don't even know what's normal now.
- My friends are getting annoyed with me talking about cancer but I'm still suffering and I can't ask for help.
- My partner just doesn't get what I'm going through.

Loneliness is a particularly hard thing to deal with. It can feel like you're not cared for and it can instil intense feelings of hurt, sadness, unworthiness and dejection. So, what can you do if you're in this position, how can you cope with these feelings of loneliness and what can you do to make your friends and family understand your position better? These are very good questions and later in this chapter Allie Morgan, a wonderful confidence coach with lots of experience in helping people cope with post-cancer challenges, is going to give her advice. However, it's worth just looking at each of these feelings in a little more detail, to understand why friends and family might be backing off.

My friends have drifted away since the end of treatment and yet it's the time when I need them most

It's not unusual for family and friends to step back from you at this point. And this is usually because their understanding is that you're no longer a cancer patient: you've been cured/you're in remission/you've beaten cancer[1] and thus you no longer need the daily and weekly support, encouragement and kindness that's directed at cancer patients.

Most of the time, this genuinely isn't a case of friends and family being intentionally unkind. There's no intended malice. It's just the way that people who haven't had cancer, can react. Why wouldn't they react in this way? They've never been in your position so they just don't know that finishing treatment brings all these other physical, emotional and mental issues and that, actually, you could still do with their support. And seeing how they've not been in your position; they can only act on how they perceive and understand the situation.

Put yourself in their shoes for a moment: in their minds you're normal again. You're one of them again. They probably think you're fine and you no longer have a need for a hand to hold, an ear to bend or a shoulder to cry on. Only cancer patients need those things and – hooray – you're no longer a cancer patient.

Nonetheless, a lack of support at a time when you most need it is terribly upsetting and can be pretty hard to deal with. Take Mary for example, she explained her situation to me:

'Throughout my treatment I had a huge amount of wonderful support from my friends. They were by my side every step of the way. But since treatment ended, my friends have backed off and this makes me so sad because this is the time when I need my friends more than ever. I need to talk to my friends about what I've just been through and how to move on. I feel really lonely at the moment. My friends and family don't understand that I need their support more than ever'.

And Ruth described her situation in this way,

'People see the end of chemo as the end of treatment. The "just checking in" messages from friends came to a stop once chemo was over but there was still so far to go'.

My friends don't understand what I'm going through

You might think that your friends and family just don't 'get' what you're going through now. Perhaps you're thinking that they don't understand:

- the anxiety I'm going through;
- how sad I feel right now;
- that calling me brave, inspirational and strong just makes me feel like a fraud as I'm none of those things;
- the fatigue I'm feeling;
- that I lie awake for hours every night thinking about the cancer coming back;
- how ugly I feel with my hair just starting to grow;
- that the treatment broke me and it's going to take a while to piece me back together;
- the all-encompassing fear of cancer coming back;
- that the diagnosis turned my world upside down and I can't seem to turn it back up the right way;
- how hard it is for me to leave the house;
- that every twinge in my body scares me;

- how jealous I am of their carefree existence;
- how lonely I feel;
- that I can't keep up with them on a night out;
- the terror I've felt for the past few months;
- everything I've just been through: the prodding, the poking, the scanning, the sleepless nights, the inability to eat, the heavy weight on my chest, the difficulty breathing, the constantly sweaty palms, the shaking, the anxiety, the worry and the fear;
- that I can't just switch off the feelings I'm currently experiencing;
- that a whole stack of new scary feelings are rearing their ugly heads now that treatment has finished;
- that I can't remember how to be normal;
- that the hard part has only just begun.

Can you relate to any of these thoughts? Well, you're certainly not the only one – the lack of understanding from friends after treatment came up time and time again during my interviews for this book. Kate told me:

'I felt really lost after treatment. The previous four months had been non-stop hospital appointments and all I'd talked about with my friends, family and colleagues had been cancer. We hadn't talked about anything else. Then when treatment ended, the cancer talk stopped – everyone assumed I was okay and people no longer asked me how I was doing – but I wasn't okay'.

Whilst Kathryn said:

'With cancer, people see the physical effect when you lose your hair. But after treatment ends, your hair grows back and people assume that it's all over but it's not. Life after cancer is only just starting and it's like living with an invisible illness'.

And Molly explained:

'Friends are great but no matter how great your support network is, as someone who's just finished cancer treatment, you're still isolated from everyone'.

Yes, it's upsetting, frustrating and galling not to be understood by those close to you, but it's perfectly normal. Unless someone has been through cancer themselves, they just can't relate to how it feels when the treatment ends and you're left to process what you've been through while adapting to life after cancer. Again, put yourself in their shoes: how would they know that you're feeling the way you are, while they're celebrating the back of cancer and waving it off into the distance?

My family and friends think my life can go back to normal but I don't even know what normal means

As I've already said, when treatment finishes, your friends and family will be elated. They will be so relieved that you're no longer a cancer patient and that you've successfully completed cancer treatment to the point where you no longer have cancer. They will certainly want to celebrate. For them, the end of treatment represents the end of cancer and signifies the point in time when they will get you, their loved one, back. To them, no more cancer treatment means you are back to normal and life can carry on from where you left it on the day of your diagnosis.

However, contrary to what friends and family might expect, we all know that getting to the end of treatment isn't like flicking a switch from cancer patient to normality. Far from it – it's why I've written this book and why you're reading this book. In fact, it's quite possible that you may be feeling the opposite to normal and it can be quite upsetting if you don't feel understood or heard by your friends and family. Take Emily for example. She explained:

> 'Now that treatment is over, I don't update my friends about what I'm going through as much as I did during my treatment. So it's not obvious that I'm going through what I'm going through. They think I'm back to normal but I'm not'.

And Jo H told me:

> 'I felt incredibly alone after treatment ended. Whilst my family and friends had been hugely supportive throughout treatment, once treatment was over the support drifted away. I guess they assumed I must be fine because I'd finished treatment and the cancer was all behind me. But it was the opposite. Finishing treatment was the hardest part for me and nobody in my life understood what I was going through'.

My friends are getting annoyed with me talking about cancer but I'm still suffering and I can't ask for help

Many people who have finished cancer treatment feel that their family and friends are so bored with the topic of cancer, that they can't talk to them about how they're feeling or what they're going through. It's common to think that your friends and family don't want to hear about cancer *again* and that they want to move on from cancer. Cathy and Mary both told me that they'd experienced this. Cathy commented:

'I was saddened by people's impatience with me and their dismissiveness when I wanted, or really needed, to talk about what happened to me'.

And Mary said:

'My friends just want me to be back to normal. Some friends have even encouraged me to move on with my life now, but I'm just not there yet. In fact, I've had to distance myself from some friends – the ones who ask me why I'm still talking about cancer. I'm so paranoid that they'll get annoyed with me. They think I need to move on, but I can't. Why can't they understand what I'm going through?'.

This is especially hard as you might end up thinking that you have to deal with this stage of the process on your own, when in actual fact you need help and support more than ever.

I feel lonely: my partner doesn't get it

It's been said by so many people at this stage of cancer recovery, that once treatment is over, it's not just friends who have an expectation that life will return to normal, but partners also have this expectation. A number of the women whom I interviewed – and who have partners – told me that they'd experienced a lack of understanding from their partners. I was told:

'My relationship suffered as well. I was angry with my partner because as soon as I'd been given the "all-clear" he thought that I should be over it'.

And someone else explained:

'My husband and son are so relieved that I'm still here after having had breast cancer but they don't understand that I'm still feeling fragile. My husband was amazing throughout treatment. Now he thinks that I'm done with cancer and that I should be happy and move on. It is like he has just drawn a line under it, it is over, move on. He doesn't understand that I'm still reeling from it'.

The difference between – on one hand – partners having this expectation and – on the other hand – friends, is that you have a higher expectation of your partner. After all, your partner has effectively lived through the cancer diagnosis and treatment with you, so obviously you're going to expect them to have a better understanding of exactly how you're feeling now that treatment has ended. And let's be honest here, sometimes we do expect our partner to be telepathic and know what's going on without us having to spell it out. It's this divergence of expectations which often can lead to conflict at home.

Coping with the loneliness

As you can see, there are many ways in which people can feel alone at this stage. When friends and family drift away at the end of treatment, Allie likens it to a marathon. She says:

> 'It can feel a bit like you've run a marathon and reached the finish line only to find that everyone has gone home. It's upsetting, disappointing and it can be difficult to know how to address this at a stage when you're experiencing so many complicated feelings and emotions'.

So, how can you deal with the loneliness? Well, Allie's first piece of advice is simple: talk to your friends and family. She says that it's important to talk to your friends and family honestly and openly about how you're feeling. They've not been where you are right now, so they genuinely don't know how you're feeling. If you can explain to them that despite finishing treatment, you're still feeling the impact of cancer then they'll understand your situation and be better placed to support you.

You might think that this will be a hard conversation to have, but cancer really shows you who your friends are so if a friend has been there for you throughout treatment, they'll most likely continue to be there for you after treatment. The important thing is to be open and honest so that friends and family can understand what you're going through and can be there for you.

A big aspect of loneliness after treatment might be that you're not invited to social events as much as before you had cancer. To be honest, this is probably because your friends think you'll be too tired or not feel up for it. But let's face it, that doesn't change the fact that it's really upsetting not to be invited out by your friends. So, talk to them. Tell them that you still want to be invited to things even if you don't always say yes or if you sometimes drop out at the last minute. Explain that you'd love to be included in all the things that you were included in before you had cancer, but because of the lingering side-effects of treatment, you might not be able to join in all the time.

Allie's second piece of advice is that if you're not sure how to broach the subject with friends and family then you may find it helps to use writing and journalling to understand your own emotions and articulate them into something that you can then discuss with them. If you can better understand yourself and what you're going through, then it'll be easier to explain your feelings and emotions to the people around you. The Toolkit at the back of the book has some tips for journalling and writing, so why not grab yourself a cup of tea and a pen, and start by using the notes page at the end of this chapter to plan out some of the things you could say.

Even when you explain to friends and family how you're feeling and they try to understand what you're going through, they still won't completely get it if they haven't been there. You can have all the love in the world directed your way, but still feel lonely. But you're not alone. You don't have to deal with this on your own. There are many people who have trodden this particular path before you and plenty who are walking it now and there are plenty of places where you can talk to people who are going through the same thing as you: cancer support centres, online cancer support services, Facebook groups, social media and support groups in person at support centres. Look for local groups specifically aimed at people who've been through cancer, for example choirs and walking groups. The important thing is to find somewhere where you can comfortably talk to others in your position: somewhere where you can reach out and say 'I'm feeling lonely' and immediately you'll find people who'll know how you're feeling.

> **Top tip**
> Talk to your friends and family openly and honestly about how you're feeling.

Checklist

Here's a recap of the key points for you to take away from this chapter.

1 Tell your friends and family about how you're feeling. Be open and honest.
2 Explain to friends that you'd like to be invited to social events even though you might not be able to make every event.

3 Use journalling and writing to help you process your emotions and articulate your feelings to help you talk to friends and family. There are some helpful writing prompts in the Toolkit at the back of the book which may help get you started.

4 Look for places where you can talk to other people who are going through what you're going through right now: cancer support centres, online cancer support services, Facebook groups, social media and support groups in person at support centres.

Notes

Use this page to plan what you could say to friends and family about how you're feeling now

12

Loss and grief

Grieving over what's been lost to cancer

'What I'm going through now feels a bit like grief. My brother died a couple of years ago and I feel like I'm going through the same thing as I did when I lost him. Except this time, I'm grieving for myself. Cancer has taken away my ability to have more children. I've lost a year with my son because while I've been going through treatment, I haven't been the mum to him that I want to be. I may have got my life back now, but in some ways, I feel like I haven't got my life back because I'm too tired to do half the things I used to do. I'm grieving for the body I used to have, and for a time when I didn't have to worry about as much as I do now'.

Tasha

The losses suffered as a result of cancer are not limited to the loss of a breast or the removal of lymph nodes. In fact, the loss suffered by a cancer patient extends so much further than body parts and, quite honestly, there can be such deep feelings of loss that you might not be able to see how you can ever get over it. But you will, and in this chapter I will take you through the different types of loss that you might be feeling and you'll see from all the personal anecdotes that these feelings of loss are, oh so common. Then we'll look at how you can cope with loss and grief, with insight and advice from Anne Crook, who is a counsellor in psycho-oncology and has a lot of experience in helping people going through these sorts of feelings. So, let's get started by looking some of the things that you might feel you've lost due to cancer.

You've lost a chunk of your life

The time during which you've been going through tests, treatment and recovery is time out of regular life that you'll never ever get back. You may have missed birthday celebrations because you were dealing with the side-effects of treatment. You may have missed your child's school play because you had a hospital appointment. You might have missed a host of social and family events because you were feeling too weak to attend.

For example, Kathryn told me:

'I mostly feel loss surrounding motherhood and time with my daughter. I look at photos of us together before cancer – having fun and going to places – and it just reminds me how much has changed. I'm not able to go out with her on my own now because I don't have the energy to look after her. I can't be the mum that I was before cancer. I feel that I've lost a whole stage of motherhood to cancer and don't know when I'll get back to the energy levels of before cancer, it is extremely frustrating'.

And Gabi commented to me:

'I had a two-week-old baby when I was diagnosed with breast cancer. The timing felt so cruel. The time during which I went through treatment is time that I'll never get back. Cancer has taken that away from me'.

Whatever it is that you've missed during the course of your treatment, it can be incredibly upsetting thinking that you've lost a chunk of your life to cancer.

You may have lost the ability to have children

Cancer treatment can cause infertility and make conceiving a child so much more challenging. Emily explained to me:

'We don't have children and it's never been on the cards for us to have children. But then I was diagnosed and one of the first things I was asked was whether we wanted to have children in which case we'd have to freeze my eggs. We didn't go down that route and even though we'd never had plans to have children, knowing that it's not even an option now is a big thing for me to deal with'.

In addition, it's usual for women who've had certain hormone related cancers, to be advised not to have a baby for a certain period after treatment. This can inevitably mean that by the time a woman on hormone therapy reaches the end of the advised period, she's too old to have a baby. Gabi and Mary are both in this situation. Gabi explained:

'I've been advised not to get pregnant for five to ten years: even in five years' time I'll be too old to have another baby, so the choice of whether to have a larger family has been taken out of my hands. Cancer's taken that away from me too'.

And Mary told me:

> 'I was lucky enough to have two rounds of egg preservation and I have 12 embryos on ice, but I still have Herceptin and Tamoxifen for a number of years. All my friends are having kids and I'm scared that I won't be able to – it's not going to be easy'.

One way or another, it's not unusual for cancer to take away the ability to have children. Infertility due to cancer treatment is such a huge issue to deal with that it really deserves specialized and professional help, which is beyond the remit of this book. If you are affected by infertility please seek professional advice, counselling and guidance.

You may have lost friends

Whilst, on the whole, many friends can be an amazing support for you during cancer, it's sadly not unusual for some friends to back away or distance themselves as you go through your treatment. Take Molly's experience for example:

> 'My friendships have been massively impacted by cancer. I was completely let down by one of my (I thought) best friends who said she would be my cancer buddy but then completely disappeared. We'd been friends for 13 years and yet she just wasn't there for me as I went through cancer'.

Natasha also experienced friendship issues. She told me:

> 'Cancer has affected my friendships. Several people I had known for years just vanished during my cancer treatment. It was hurtful and very lonely'.

It's a bitter pill to swallow when this happens, but it happens and it happens for a variety of reasons. Some people might feel uncomfortable around someone with cancer – they might not know how to act or what to say or what to do around you and instead of telling you this they find it easier to just back off. Some people might be reminded of a time that someone close to them went through cancer and they can't face watching someone else go through it. Some people might be going through some tricky times themselves – perhaps going through some personal issues of their own which you know nothing about. And of course, someone who isn't there for you during cancer treatment might, sadly, just not be the good friend that you thought they were.

Whatever the reason for their absence, the sad reality is that you can lose friends through cancer and it is completely and utterly heart breaking. Mary told me:

'While I was going through cancer treatment, some of my friends who'd I expected to be there for me, were not there for me. Yes, there was a lot of surface support with comments like, "it's all going to be ok" and "you are strong, you will fight this", but not the deeper support that I really needed from these friends. Sadly, I've had to distance myself from these people because it hurts that they couldn't be there for me when I needed them the most'.

You may have lost opportunities at work

It's very common for people to take time off work during cancer treatment. The treatment can be so intense and the side-effects so all-consuming that it's just impossible to maintain a normal working life. But unfortunately, despite the legal obligations placed on employers to protect employees with cancer, it's inevitable that missing time at work can lead to missed opportunities, such as a promotion, getting a new contract or heading up a new project.

Amy lost many work opportunities during the year she went through breast cancer treatment. She explained:

'I work in television production and it's all contract work. I was a Production Secretary and was looking to step up to Production Coordinator in the near future. But then I got breast cancer and had to take a significant amount of time off work so instead of being promoted to Production Coordinator, I remained at the Production Secretary level'.

And for those who are self-employed, it can be incredibly challenging keeping the business going whilst going through treatment whether due to the inability to physically keep running the business or the mental toll of cancer treatment leading to a lack of motivation and enthusiasm. Take Kathryn, for example, who explained:

'I used to be a reiki healer for horses but I can't go back to doing that because I don't have the physical energy or the emotional capacity. I'm not sure if I will ever. I've lost my enthusiasm for it – it was a big part of who I was and not sure if I will ever get back to it'.

And Lindsey, whose experience was:

> 'I used to have a part time cake decorating business but I had to close the business during treatment and I haven't been able to restart it due to the peripheral neuropathy and fatigue'.

You may have lost a part of yourself

Have you seen a photograph of yourself before cancer and been saddened by the loss of that person? I certainly felt that way and this came up a lot in the conversations I had with the women for this book. Molly said to me:

> 'I look at photos from a couple of years and I think, "who is that person? Is that really me?". The woman in the photos was innocent and didn't know the horrors of cancer and cancer treatment'.

And Cathy commented:

> 'For a while after treatment, I didn't want to think about the old me and I got upset when looking back at the photos of me before cancer. I miss her'.

There's something in that pre-cancer version of yourself that doesn't exist now isn't there? Perhaps it's an innocence or a naivety: the way that person lived their life not knowing that something so awful could happen to them. Perhaps it's the blissful, carefree existence they lead in that photo, not realizing that life isn't always easy but can throw some pretty serious punches at times. Or perhaps it's an arrogant belief that they're invincible and assume that life will carry on the way it always has for them.

This feeling – that you've lost a part of yourself – is, hands down, one of the most common feelings experienced by people who go through cancer. Gabi told me:

> 'Prior to my diagnosis I lived in a little bubble where things like cancer just didn't happen. I lived my life with the attitude that something like cancer "won't happen to me". I realize now that I was living a slightly naive existence. But in a way it's good that people are living like this because you don't want everyone wondering around worrying about dying. But once you experience something that makes you realize that you could have died, it means that you then have to learn to live with the fact that death from cancer is actually a real possibility and doesn't just happen to other people. I miss my naivety and my "isn't life wonderful" attitude'.

And Emily explained:

> 'Right now, I think I'm struggling with the loss of my pre-cancer life, the loss of the feeling that I'm untouchable. The loss of being just a normal friend, not the one friend that had cancer'.

Whatever it is in that photo of pre-cancer you – or in the memory of the pre-cancer you – it's hard to accept that you can't go back to that person knowing what you now know and having been through what you've been through.

You may have lost part of your identity

Some of you may feel like you've lost part of your identity. You may have had a mastectomy and lost one or both breasts, you may have lost the use of another part of your body, or you may have lost your hair, eyelashes and eyebrows. All of which – in your mind – form part of your identity. Take Juliet for example, who explained to me:

> 'I had a single mastectomy without reconstruction and it had such a huge impact on me that I insisted on having a mastectomy on the other side and I now live flat. After my initial mastectomy, I was really disturbed by the space left from the removal of my breast whilst on the other side I still had a breast. The remaining breast represented who I was, whilst the space on the other side represented the future me and the two didn't work together side by side. I realized that I would have to lose my other breast to move forward as the new version of me'.

And Emily, who said:

> 'I recently had a big cry as I realized that I felt a huge sense of loss about my body and who I was before cancer'.

When losing something so integral to yourself and your identity, the loss can feel enormous. Looking in the mirror can be a distressing experience and this can cause a loss of confidence in the future. Remember that there's some advice about adjusting to these aspects of loss in Chapter 9 which covers how to adjust to changes to your physical appearance.

You may have lost a social life

Your social circles don't stop going out and having fun just because you're laid up with cancer. And sadly, due to innumerable side-effects, overwhelming fatigue and perhaps a lack of confidence, you might have found yourself missing more social occasions than you actually managed to make. After constantly having to turn down social invitations during treatment, some of you might even have found social invitations have dried up by the time you get to the end of treatment and you've reached a time when you'd like to start going out and seeing people again.

It can be incredibly hard to experience this sort of thing. One of the women I interviewed for this book told me:

> 'I definitely missed out on social events during my treatment. I was told by friends that they didn't think I'd want to come. That hurt.'

Sadly, this sort of comment is not unusual.

Coping with the loss

Oh my, there really is so much to lose when you go through cancer treatment. When something important is lost, it's natural to grieve for that loss. This is why, when you reach the end of treatment and you start to process what you've been through, it can feel like you're grieving for something. Which – on top of everything else you're going through – can feel really rather discombobulating. So, with Anne's help, insight and advice let's look at coping with loss and grief

According to Anne, feelings of loss, and the consequential grief for those losses, is completely normal after cancer. And yet, some of you might not even realize that the sadness or emptiness that you're feeling is down to loss. Only after sitting with the sadness for a while, will you recognize that you've lost something. But before we get to how exactly you can sit with the sadness and recognize that you're grieving, let's just recap for a moment. Let's look at everything you've been through in order to understand where you are now.

After the initial mind-blowing shock of being diagnosed with cancer you were thrown – no, catapulted – into an entirely new way of life. Whilst trying to get your head around a heck of a lot of new information, your body was subjected to treatment – possibly causing unpleasant, painful or distressing side-effects. During treatment, all your emotional resources were – rightly and appropriately – focused on survival and doing what you had to do in order to get through treatment and come out the other end. Your life was structured by appointments and your treatment regime, and you will have had to make a lot of changes to your day-to-day life. As you've read time and time again in this book – it's only now, at the end of active treatment as the dust begins to settle, that the emotional impact of what you've been through hits home. It's now that you have the capacity to think about it and the space to notice the feelings that you're experiencing. You may not be *actively* reflecting on what you've been through or how you feel now, but just having the time and space allows you to become aware of emotions and feelings that perhaps weren't noticeable until now.

With this time and space to notice your emotions and feelings it's now that the emotional processing can begin. It's often at this point when people are taken by surprise that contrary to what they'd expected throughout treatment – that they'd get back to normal after treatment – they don't actually return to the same person in the life they had before cancer. And with this shock realization that you're not going to be the same person or have the same life as you did before cancer, comes the realization of what you've lost: the missing and longing for what cancer may have taken from you, and the need to mourn and grieve for this.

And, according to Anne, this is the first step in dealing with the loss and grief associated with your cancer experience: the recognition of the loss, or losses, that you've suffered and the recognition that life doesn't feel the same any more but that something needs to happen before you can adjust to where you are now. There needs to be a conscious emotional process by which you can acknowledge the losses and what has gone.

Let's simplify things here – Anne suggests that it might help you to imagine your life as a jigsaw puzzle. As you're doing the puzzle over the course of your life – putting the pieces together – the picture of your life is forming. There's your family, there's your career or job, over there are your friends and down there are your interests. Then cancer arrives and the pieces of the jigsaw are scattered everywhere. You try to pick up the pieces in order to put them back together but every piece you pick up seems to be about cancer and cancer is taking over the picture. But now, after treatment has finished, there are less pieces about cancer and you can get on with putting the puzzle back together. But as you're doing this you notice that not only is the picture not the same picture as before, but there are also missing pieces. The things that you've lost.

Although it might not feel like it right now, it is perfectly possible to rebuild this jigsaw. It will take some work on your part and the picture won't be the same as it was prior to the arrival of cancer in your life, but you'll gradually fill in the gaps with new pieces and you'll see new images appear in the picture. And to help you do this, Anne's advice is:

- Understand that it's normal to feel loss as you begin your recovery.
- Become aware of, and acknowledge, what you've lost.
- Recognize that something has gone and either you might not get it back at all, or you might get some of it back but it'll be back in a different way. Your hair might grow back differently, you may have a different circle of close friends, you might find that you'd rather read a book than go out on a night out, or you may find that your priorities in life have changed.
- It's important to mourn the losses. Allow yourself to acknowledge that you miss the person you were before cancer and the life you had before cancer. Allow yourself to feel sad about this and acknowledge that it might be helpful for you to talk to someone about how you are feeling. In talking to someone about how you're feeling, it's important to talk to someone who will allow you to talk and listen to what you say. You need to be heard and not dismissed. And you don't need your listener to try to fix everything. You could talk to someone with whom you are close and who is a good listener, someone who has had cancer and been through what you're going through, or a professional counsellor.
- It can be helpful to read the accounts of other people who've been through the same thing that you've been through and from which you'll recognize aspects of your own experience. It's always comforting knowing that you're not the only one who feels a certain way.
- You don't need to go through a long period of mourning, but you need to give what you're feeling some kind of recognition in order to move on and integrate the experience of cancer into your life. There is no timetable for grief – there isn't a set way and it will take as long as it takes. Don't put pressure on yourself.
- Note that grief is a dynamic process and you won't get over all your losses at once. Over time, as you continue to process the sadness at what you've lost and as your life moves on, your feelings will change. The jigsaw puzzle will start to fit back together; there'll be fewer pieces

associated with cancer; some of the old parts of the jigsaw will come back into focus; and where there were gaps, you'll start filling with new pieces.

- Recognize that you may have lost some things, but you've also gained some things – try listing all the gains or opportunities that you've made during cancer, such as new friends, a strength you didn't know you had and an appreciation for the important things in life.
- You could try writing and journalling about your experience with a focus on the things you've lost and how you are mourning for them. People also find it cathartic to write poetry to express their experience.
- Try creating some rituals around your grief, for example you could take all the cancer information sheets that you were handed when diagnosed and dump them in the recycling; you could donate all the lounging clothes that you wore throughout treatment to charity; or you could write a letter saying goodbye to everything you've lost.

Top tip

The first step in grieving for what you've lost through cancer is recognizing that life doesn't feel the same anymore and that something needs to happen before you can adjust to where you are now.

Checklist

Here's a recap of the key points for you to take away from this chapter.

1 Understand that it's normal to feel loss after going through cancer treatment.
2 Try to recognize what you've lost.
3 Try to acknowledge that life doesn't feel the same anymore and that something needs to happen before you can adjust to where you are now.
4 It's important to mourn your losses. Allow yourself to feel sad and to miss the person you were before cancer. It can help to talk to someone – whether a good friend or professional counsellor – about how you're feeling.
5 Know that you're allowed to feel sad about the things you've lost.

6 If it doesn't trigger anxiety in you, it can be helpful to read accounts of other people who are going through what you're going through, to understand that you are not alone in feeling this way.

7 Understand that grief takes as long as it takes and over time your feelings will change.

8 Recognize any gains you've made: friendships, a new outlook on life or a re-evaluation of the important things in your life.

9 Writing and journalling can help express your feelings of loss and grief. The Toolkit at the back of the book includes some advice and writing prompts to get you started.

Notes

Use this page to express your feelings about what you've lost through cancer.

13

Loss of confidence

Coping with the loss of confidence after cancer

'I've really lost my confidence since treatment: I have a big dent in one of my breasts; I lost my hair, eyelashes and eyebrows during chemo; I put on weight during treatment and now when I look in the mirror, I feel unattractive. I'm in my twenties and engaged to be married so I should be feeling my best but I feel far from it'.

Mary

There's a big loss that wasn't covered in the previous chapter – the loss of self-confidence. This is such a significant loss, and one which can hinder day-to-day life while you're trying to move forward after treatment. So, I'm dedicating an entire chapter on how to cope with a loss of self-confidence and regain your self-confidence (note that the issue of body confidence after cancer is covered in Chapter 9).

But first, let me tell you that it's important to note that losing your self-confidence as a result of cancer is perfectly normal. There's something about going through cancer treatment that can instil a vulnerability and lower your confidence. Maybe it's the need for help in many areas of life during treatment, a side-effect of anxiety or the inability to do some of the day-to-day basics as a result of fatigue. But whatever the cause, for many people, their confidence can fly out the window following a cancer diagnosis and it doesn't just reappear when treatment ends.

Take Kathryn, for example, who explained to me;

'I've not gone back to work yet. I work for the local council and I'm really anxious about going back to work. A big part of the job is dealing with people on the phone and I have to deal with some difficult issues. I don't think that I'm emotionally up to dealing with this sort of thing yet and I don't know when I will be'.

Whilst Jo H summed up how she was feeling by telling me:

'I've suffered from feelings of really low self-worth'.

According to Allie Morgan (the Confidence Coach who provided insight and advice earlier in Chapter 11) it's perfectly normal to reach the end of treatment and feel like you've lost your confidence. You've been through a hell of a lot and so why wouldn't a big chunk of confidence fly out the window? Now that treatment is over, you can start to rebuild your confidence as well as your physical strength. And a big part of rebuilding your confidence is learning to love yourself again.

Allie's advice is to start by addressing your relationship with your body. You might feel like your body has let you down by allowing the cancer to grow. You might not like the way you look now: your hair may be different, you may not have eyebrows or eyelashes, you may have put on weight or lost weight, you may have scars, you may have changes to your body if you've had surgery and you may be battling the fatigue on a daily basis. The way you feel about your body has a real impact on your confidence. Take Jo H for example. She said to me:

> 'Cancer has definitely affected my body confidence: I don't like how my breast feels and I think my husband no longer finds me attractive because of it'.

So, now is the time to address your relationship with your body. Allie says:

> 'Learn to appreciate everything that your body has been through. It's been through a hell of a lot and yet here it is: it's still working and actually it's done an amazing job of getting you to the here and now. Yes, it may have allowed cancer to grow within you, and yes you may look and feel physically different as a result of treatment, but your body has withstood a real battering from the onslaught of surgery, anaesthetics, chemotherapy drugs, radiation and more. Be patient with it. Allow it to recover in time. Don't push the exercise, don't force the hair regrowth, don't fight the weight gain. Take it slowly. Be kind to your body and yourself. Be aware of the way you speak to yourself. As humans, we naturally focus on negative thoughts. It's just the way our brains work. So, now is the time to focus on positive thoughts and to learn to love yourself again'.

I know it's all very well hearing that you need to learn to love yourself again, but you're probably wondering how, in reality, can you do that? Well, to get you started on loving yourself again and rebuilding your confidence, Allie is sharing her top tips:

- Become aware of how you're talking to yourself and treating yourself. Are you putting yourself down with thoughts such as: I'm ugly without hair; I'm too tired and my face is too puffy; nobody wants me around as I'm too tired; I won't be any good when I go back to work because I won't remember how to do my job? Lots of people don't think that they are worthy enough for lots of things after cancer. Is this how you would speak to your best friend or a beloved family member? No? Well then, don't talk to yourself like this. Being aware of the way you think about yourself is a huge step in turning your thoughts around.

- Now you need to introduce more positive thoughts about yourself. This might sound difficult but there are some things you can do to help this and with more practice this will feel more natural.
  - ○ Start with some daily affirmations. These are things that you can say to yourself over and over again until you believe it. So, for example, you could say *I am enough* a few times every morning when you wake up and a few times at the end of the day as you're going to bed. You might feel a bit silly saying these things to yourself, but soon it won't feel so silly. Using positive affirmations can actually change your habit of thinking negatively. The Toolkit at the back of the book contains a section on affirmations and some suggested affirmations that you can use.
  - ○ Try practising a gratitude exercise on a daily basis when you get up in the morning: look in the mirror and name one thing for which you are grateful, one thing that you love about yourself and one thing that you're working on.
  - ○ Next is to think about the way you treat yourself. Be kind to yourself. Practise self-care. Take a nap if you need to. Make yourself delicious, healthy food. Do some exercise that you enjoy. Get some fresh air. If you were taking care of a friend in your position, what would you do for them? You need to treat yourself the way you treat people you love.
  - ○ A lot of people measure their self-worth by what they think other people think of them. For example: *my partner probably finds me really unattractive now that I've had a mastectomy; my colleagues will resent me for having so much time off work; my friends will think I'm boring as I'm tired all the time.* Don't do this, it's really not very helpful at all and can be quite damaging to your self-confidence. Work on your self-belief. Cancer is only part of your story, it's not the entire story. It's just a part of you, making you who you are. It's

not what defines you. Talk to your friends about how you're feeling. Explain that whilst you're not yet over cancer and it'll take a bit of time, you don't want their opinion of you to change. Remember that good friends will be there for you and they'll understand.

Top tip
Don't measure your self-worth by what you think other people think about you.

Checklist

Here's a recap of the key points for you to take away from this chapter.

1 Know that it's perfectly normal to reach the end of treatment and feel like you've lost a big chunk of your self-confidence.
2 Learn to appreciate your body and to be grateful to it for getting you to the here and now.
3 Be patient with your body's recovery.
4 Talk to yourself as you would talk to someone you love.
5 Use daily affirmations to think more positively about yourself.
6 Treat yourself as kindly as you would treat a good friend.
7 Practise self-care and be kind to yourself.
8 Recognize that it is a normal way of thinking to measure your self-worth by what others think of you – but it's unhelpful and not based on truth. Bring yourself back to the truth and what you know which is that you are NOT useless, boring, ugly or unlikeable.
9 Talk to your friends and family to explain how you're feeling and that you don't want their opinion of you to change now that you've had cancer.

Notes

Use this page to record some positive things about yourself; write some daily affirmations and make notes about the things for which you are grateful

14

Trusting your body after cancer

How can you trust your body again after it's let you down in such a big way?

Dear body,

I trusted you and you've let me down. Let me down badly.

How did you allow a cancerous tumour to grow inside me? Which, I now find out, had been growing for quite a while!

I didn't know that you were hiding cancer from me until it had grown to a point where it couldn't hide any longer. How could you do that to me?

I've looked after you my whole life, so why have you done this? Do all those healthy meals and exercise mean nothing to you?

Why didn't you let me know something was wrong earlier so I could fix it without all the horrible cancer treatment?

How can I trust you again if you tried to kill me?

Where do we go from here? I don't want to break up with you but I can't see how to rebuild the trust.

Kind regards,

Person who's had cancer

Does this sound familiar? If so, you're most definitely not the only one. Take Rachel L, for example, who told me:

'I've definitely lost trust in my body – having cancer really shook my confidence in my body. I feel that I didn't do enough to support my body before I got cancer, and although I've since made changes to my lifestyle, I don't trust that I won't get cancer again'.

Whilst Ruth explained:

'I have no trust in my body. I feel like it's failed me, and now I feel like I'm failing mentally. I have no faith in myself physically in the long run'.

It's certainly not unusual to question the trust in your body after having been through cancer, but why is this and how can you deal with these feelings of mistrust?

Let's start by looking at the trust we place in our bodies. Whilst we might take our bodies for granted, a lot of what we do on a daily basis is aimed at keeping them healthy. Take a typical day, we sleep to rest the body and allow it to rejuvenate and recover; we eat to feed it the nutrients it needs to able to fight off illnesses; we exercise to stay in good shape inside and out; and most of us try to limit the bad things like smoking, alcohol and stress in order to give our bodies the best chance of remaining fit, strong and healthy.

It's a two-way thing – you might even say it's a relationship in some ways. By doing all these things to look after our bodies, in return we expect something back. We trust that our bodies will work properly and won't let us down.

But getting cancer can feel like your body has let you down. You didn't know that cancer was growing inside you until you noticed a change and you realized something wasn't quite right. In the case of breast cancer, it might have been a lump that wasn't there the last time you looked; it might have been a change in the shape of your breast that you hadn't previously noticed; or it might have been a change in the texture of the skin of your breast that seemed to appear from nowhere. Or you might not even have noticed something yourself: for some people, their cancer is not found by them but rather by a routine screening appointment such as a mammogram.

Different cancers grow at different rates. Some cancers grow slowly, whilst others grow quite quickly. But regardless of how long it took for the cancer to grow in your body, it's freaking scary to think of something growing inside you, the existence of which you were blissfully unaware – perhaps even for some time.

It's quite often at this point in time – now that the busy period of treatment is over – that you might start to question how you can trust your body after it let you down by allowing the cancer to grow within you. You might be asking yourself things like:

- How the hell could all this have been going on – quite literally under my nose – without me knowing it? How could my body do this to me? How can I possibly trust my body now?

- How on earth could my body allow those mutant cells to go unnoticed for so long?
- How did my body allow those mutant cells to develop into a cancerous tumour in the first place?
- Why didn't I know that something wasn't working properly in my body?
- How could I have had the worst disease in the entire world and not have felt ill?
- Why weren't the cancerous cells destroyed by the immune system long before they had the chance to grow into a tumour?
- What about all the exercise and healthy eating that I do?
- How can I trust my body now? How can I trust that it will do its job at destroying mutant cells before they become cancerous?
- How can I trust my body to tell me something is wrong earlier on?
- How can I trust something that tried to kill me – how do I know it won't do that again?
- How can I trust my body to remain healthy and not to get ill from something else?

Those are a lot of questions to get your head around at this point. However, all those questions come down to three issues.

The first issue is the question of why you got cancer in the first place. We've looked at the issue of *Why me?* in Chapter 6 so head back there for a reminder of how to deal with this way of thinking. The second issue is that of it happening again – that the cancer will return. We looked at the fear of recurrence in Chapter 5 so head back there to revisit the advice about coping with a fear of the cancer coming back. The third issue is what we're looking at in this chapter: it's the question of trust in your body. How you can get back to a place where you can go about daily life, relying on your body to do its job and to do it properly – fighting off illnesses, getting rid of any mutant cells and letting you know when there's a problem that needs to be looked into.

Like I said earlier, let's think of it as a relationship. We put in the work to look after our bodies and we expect something in return – we expect our bodies to do their job at expelling the bad stuff and giving us a heads up when things aren't quite right. With cancer, our bodies haven't expelled the bad stuff and it might feel like a heads-up about something not being right was given quite late in the day, especially if the cancer cells had spread to the lymph nodes and you required chemotherapy.

It's really important to rebuild the trust in your body. Firstly, if you can rebuild the trust in your body then maybe you won't be questioning every twinge, ache or pain as a possible recurrence of cancer. Maybe it will help allow you to live your daily life without constantly second guessing everything that is going on in your body. Maybe you'll be able to get back the faith that your body will look after you. Secondly, it's important to rebuild the trust because cancer isn't the only risk you face: there are also the same risks that everyone else faces and you have to learn to trust that your body will keep working against all potential threats, whether that's the common cold or something more serious. And thirdly, it's important to get back to a place of trust so that you look after your body as well as you can. When the trust is no longer in a relationship, there is a risk of the betrayed party not treating the betraying party well. Perhaps you're thinking that your body didn't look after you so why should you look after it? Why should you eat a healthy diet, why should you exercise and why should you avoid all the bad stuff? Building back the trust in your body will encourage you to do your best to look after your body. You can go back to treating it with love and kindness: treating it well in the knowledge that it will do its best to remain healthy.

Rebuilding the trust

So how do we build up the trust again? How do we get over this betrayal? Rebuilding the trust in your body won't happen overnight. It's a gradual process and it will require some work on your part, but it can be achieved. To help rebuild the trust, here's some helpful advice from Allie Morgan (who has provided insight and advice in some of the earlier chapters). Why not get yourself a drink, have a read of Allie's advice and make some notes on the notes page at the end of this chapter.

Treat your body well

- Like any relationship where there has been a breakdown of trust, understand that it might take a while to rebuild the trust so be patient and give it time.
- Be compassionate and kind to your body. Treat it well by eating healthy, nutritious meals, exercising and practising self-care.

Get to know your body again

- Your body may well have changed since cancer so it's important to reconnect with your body as it is now. Start off by taking small steps at getting to know your body again. Maybe treat yourself to a nice moisturizer and after your shower or bath, spend some time getting to know your body again. Can you start to think of every part of your body as being something to cherish? Think of yourself as the queen of your body and all the cells in your body as the people in your kingdom. When you pay attention to part of your body, all the cells in that part of the body will be lining the street waiting for the queen to visit.
- If your physical appearance has changed as a result of cancer treatment, it can be difficult to come to terms with some of the changes, and this may hinder your ability to rebuild the trust in your body. Chapter 8 provides advice on coping with physical changes so it's worth referring back there if this applies to you.

Don't forget that your body is just part of your person

- It can help to look at yourself as four parts: the physical part, the emotional part, the spiritual part and the mental health part. Rebuilding the trust in your body involves all four parts of you and giving attention to all of these parts will help rebuild the trust.
- For example, to tend to the physical body you can exercise, eat healthily and avoid smoking; to tend to your emotional needs you could talk to a friend or write about your feelings; to tend to your spiritual side you could meditate or visit your place of worship; and to tend to your mental health you could do something for your mind such as using art therapy to explore the trust you have in your body.
- Try to focus on one area a day so that you are not constantly focusing on the body, but rather yourself as a person.

Increasing your body confidence can help to rebuild your trust in your body

- Wear clothes that make you feel good and build your confidence.
- Try to appreciate and love your body the way it is, for example look at your scars as things to appreciate rather than hide.

- Avoid comparing your body to others, especially on social media. It's very easy to compare your body to others but this is incredibly unhelpful and unhealthy. Everyone's body is unique to them – everyone has a different bone structure, different metabolism, different cells and different genes – so there is no point in comparing how you look with how someone else looks.

Show gratitude to your body

- Reframe the way that you look at your body. Instead of blaming your body for getting cancer, maybe it's time to thank your body for all that it has done for you?
- For those of you who found out something was wrong outside of a routine screening, remember that even though you didn't know that a malignant tumour was growing to start with, at some point your body told you that something wasn't right. Whether it was the breast lump or some other sign, at some point your body communicated that there was something wrong and you were able to get it checked out. And it was down to that communication that you're here right now.
- And think about the way your body has rejuvenated, recovered and regenerated. Look at how your scars have healed over, look at how your radiation blisters are healing, look at how your hair is growing back and look how far you've come physically from the days when you were mid-treatment and were so fatigued and ill with side-effects from treatment. Isn't it amazing how your body can heal itself after all of that?
- Try incorporating gratitude for your body in your writing and journalling. Maybe you could think of – and write about – one thing that you are grateful to your body for every day.

> Dear body,
>
> Thank you.
>
> I know I don't say this very often, but thank you for everything that you do for me.
>
> Thank you for doing your job and trying to fight the mutant cancer cells. I know you did your best, but they were just too determined to grow. Thank you for notifying me when they got out of control.

Thank you for getting me through all the treatment: for recovering, rejuvenating and regenerating after all the surgery, chemotherapy and radiotherapy.

Thank you for getting me to today and taking me to tomorrow.

Kind regards,

Person who's moving on from cancer

Top tip

Don't forget all the brilliant things that your body has done, like recovering, rejuvenating and regenerating.

Checklist

Here's a recap of the key points for you to take away from this chapter.

1 The issue of trust in your body can involve asking why you got cancer in the first place. Chapter 6 provides some insight and advice in relation to this issue.
2 If the question of trust in your body concerns a fear of the cancer coming back, it would be worth referring to Chapter 5 which deals with the fear of recurrence.
3 Understand that rebuilding the trust in your body is a gradual process and will not happen overnight.
4 Treat your body well, with kindness and compassion.
5 Get to know your body and how it has changed since cancer treatment.
6 Remember that your body is just part of your person and that it's important to address the physical, emotional, spiritual and mental health parts of yourself.
7 Increasing your body confidence can help to rebuild the trust in your body.
8 Be grateful to your body and remember the ways in which it has rejuvenated, recovered and regenerated since your cancer diagnosis.
9 Keeping a gratitude journal can help you focus appreciation on your body. The Toolkit at the back of the book has guidance on keeping a gratitude journal.

Notes

Use this page to make notes on rebuilding the trust in your body – how are you grateful to your body?

15

The impact of your cancer on your family

Understanding and coping with the impact of your cancer on your family

'While I was going through cancer, I thought that my three children handled it very well. But in the couple of years since treatment ended, two of my children needed help with mental health issues and I'm sure that seeing me go through cancer has been a contributing factor in this. Life didn't go back to normal for any of us after the end of my cancer treatment and maybe being a couple of years older now, has meant that they now realize the magnitude of what I went through. I also think that they worry that I'm going to get ill again'.

Rachel L.

Having cancer is like throwing a stone into a lake: there's often a ripple effect reaching out from the patient to their family around them. Cancer doesn't just impact the patient; it inevitably impacts everyone in the family, especially their partner and their children. So, just as you are now – at the end of treatment – reeling from the cancer bombshell that has just exploded in your life, so may the rest of your family. It's worth noting here that like everything else with cancer, everyone is different and not all families will be affected in the same way. Some families will come out of treatment with the partner and children pretty much unscathed by the whole episode, whilst other families will feel as if a large tornado has just blown through their lives, turning everything in its path upside down.

Regardless of how you think your cancer has impacted those around you, it's always sensible to keep an eye on the family. Without making a big deal, just be aware of changes in behaviour, increased anxiety or stress that might be down to your cancer diagnosis. Then, as and when this arises, you can take steps to deal with it.

Keeping an eye on the family for such signs can be really rather tricky for some people. Someone who comes out of cancer treatment feeling overwhelmed and consumed by the experience may find it hard to look out for signs of distress from other members of the family – because, let's face it, it can be hard enough coping with your own issues from cancer let alone noticing how it's affected those around you. It's therefore helpful to ask other members of the family – like grandparents – and good friends to help you keep an eye on the rest of your family.

In this chapter we're going to look at the potential impact of a cancer diagnosis upon your partner and relationship, but first let's look at how a cancer diagnosis can affect your children. We're going to be talking about children up to the age of around eighteen but adult children can also be badly impacted by their parent's cancer. For example, Cathy told me:

> 'I know that me having cancer had a huge impact on my grown-up daughter. She was there for me every step of the way, but after my treatment ended, she sought some counselling, which has really helped her'.

The impact on the children

So, let's talk about the kids. It's bad enough that cancer has impacted your mental and emotional health, but for it to also have had a detrimental impact on your children makes the whole cancer thing 100 per cent worse.

There is such a lot to say about the impact of a parent's diagnosis on a child that it's impossible to cover everything here. However, there are plenty of specialist books, websites and charities that can help. I've popped some recommendations in the Useful Resources section at the back of the book. But for the purpose of this book, we have the insight and advice of Barbara Babcock, who is a Coach and Trainee Family Therapist (you'll remember Barbara from Chapters 3 and 6 where she respectively provided her advice in relation to the loss of the safety net and how to cope with the why me? question). Barbara is going to explain how children may be affected by their parent's cancer, and then she's going to provide some all-important advice on what to do to help them.

How children might be impacted

So, the first question is how might children be affected by their parent's cancer? What sorts of things should you be keeping your eyes open for? According to Barbara, the impact of your cancer diagnosis will depend on the ages and emotional maturity of your children, what the children are told, what the children think is going on, and what they pick up from the rest of the family. It also depends upon what the children pick up from TV commercials (such as the cancer charity fundraiser commercials), TV programmes, films (especially the ones where the mother has died of cancer), the internet and from their friends at school – some of whom may have experienced cancer in their families. Children can experience emotions such as:

- Fear
- Anxiety
- Confusion
- Stress
- Sadness
- Anger

In addition, Barbara notes that your child might be affected by your cancer diagnosis in one of the following ways (but note that all children react differently). First of all, depending on the age and maturity of the child, a child might worry that their parent is going to die from cancer. This sort of fear doesn't usually kick until around the age of five to seven years old.[1] They may have watched films, read books or known someone whose parent had died. Fearing the death of a parent is a huge emotional issue for a child to deal with.

Secondly, seeing a parent go through treatment and the side-effects of treatment can be a real shock for a child. A parent who is usually active and hands-on might be laid up in bed with fatigue and sickness. A parent who is usually running around multi-tasking a million things might not be able to walk further than the end of the garden after surgery. And a parent might be wrapped in post-surgical bandages with post-surgical drains attached to parts of their body and lose all their hair, eyelashes and eyebrows due to chemotherapy. A child can notice all of these changes and be impacted by them.

And thirdly, the disruption to normal day-to-day life due to a parent going through cancer treatment, can be incredibly stressful on children. After all, children rely on routine and normality. With a parent going through treatment, family life can be turned upside down and everything that they associate with normality may change: someone else may take them to and from school; their parent may not be at home as much as usual and when they are at home they may be resting more; parents' roles may change with one parent doing more of the things that the other parent usually does; there may be fewer visitors to the house and fewer opportunities for visits to other families; they may have to stop going to their clubs and extracurricular activities if hospital appointments or side-effects get in the way of these; and having a parent stay overnight in hospital can be scary and upsetting.

It's very common for children to be impacted by the cancer of a parent. In researching this book, I had so many people tell me about the ways in which their children were affected. I've included a few anecdotes – from the women I interviewed – here, because I really want you to understand that you are not, by any means, alone in what you're going through.

'As a parent I worry a lot about the impact of my cancer on my children. My four-year-old son was having a lot of emotional outbursts, he appeared anxious at times and was having difficulty expressing and regulating his emotions. We took him for play therapy a year after I finished treatment. He attended six sessions of play therapy and during that period the therapist helped him learn how to express his emotions'.

Natasha

'My daughter was 15 when I went through breast cancer. Talking to her about such a difficult situation, whilst she was going through such big life changes herself, was so difficult for her'.

Gloria

'My youngest daughter, who was five when I was diagnosed, was affected so much by my cancer, and still is to this day. She had health anxiety and developed a fear of being ill. She struggled to manage her feelings and there was a lot of anger. We received counselling for her'.

Vicky

How to help your children

So, now you know what you're looking out for, how can you help them? What should you do if you notice anything concerning? Barbara's first key message is that each child is individual and the way they react to a parent's cancer diagnosis and treatment will depend on many different factors. The important thing in relation to your child's well-being is to establish whether you need to seek professional help for them. Do make a point of talking to them and understanding how they're feeling and what they're thinking.

Her second key message it that it's really important to respond sensitively to the feelings and emotions behind what your child is saying. You may need to help them name their emotions and feelings and what they are angry/scared/worried about. Helping a child name their emotions and feelings validates them and the child's experience of them, which is a very good thing for their current and future mental health. You doing this with your child teaches them how to do it themselves. Your child may be worried that you will be upset with them for how they are feeling so it's important to reassure them that this isn't the case.

Ignoring or denying your child's feelings, emotions and experiences can have a negative impact on their long-term mental health. Parents can inadvertently do this when their intentions are good. For example, a parent may not want their child to ever be upset so they do whatever they can to end the difficult episode causing the upset. But this can end up teaching the child to dismiss, repress or deny their own emotions, which isn't great for their long-term mental health. Gosh, this is a minefield, isn't it? Thankfully Barbara has some very helpful practical tips:

- Provide a space for your child to talk about their feelings. If you're finding it hard to cope with managing your child's emotions and fears in addition to your own post-cancer emotions, is there someone else that your child can talk to? Your partner, a grandparent, an aunt, an uncle or a good family friend? Remember the saying: 'It takes a village to raise a child'. Well, this is where that village can really step up.

- Try to spend some one-to-one time with each child as and when this is feasible. What you do will differ by age. It may be that you just have cuddle time on the sofa watching a favourite TV programme or reading a favourite book. This is a subtle way of providing reassurance to your child that you are present now, that you love them and that you're there for them.

- Think about ways by which you can provide subtle reassurance to your child? Draw them a quick picture and leave it on their pillow. Get heart shaped post-it notes, write a message and give it to your child as they pass by. Do things together that you used to do before cancer – this will help reassure them that life is getting back to normal for them.

- Having regular family meetings can be a good place to encourage the children to talk openly about their feelings. You could set some time aside once a week or once a month, perhaps over dinner or after dinner, at which the family is encouraged to talk about anything on their minds: what's going well, any challenges family members are experiencing and how to deal with challenges. For younger children, it can help to incorporate 'hold the spoon' whereby only the person holding the spoon is allowed to speak. This can enable everyone's voices to be heard, and for everyone to be reassured that they have been heard.
- Talk to your child's school about what's going on so that they can keep an eye on your child whilst he/she is at school and observe if there are any changes in their behaviour. Their school may also have some form of counselling service that can help your child process what they're going through.
- Older, adult children, can naturally be impacted by your cancer diagnosis and the post-treatment stage can result in a lot of difficult emotions coming to the surface for them. It's worth trying to have an open conversation (or conversations) with them about this and encouraging them to seek any help they may need at this stage – whether that is from a professional, by reading some self-help books or talking to good friends.

The impact on your partner

Now let's talk about partners. For partners, the impact upon them of watching their loved one go through cancer can be far reaching and, quite frankly, a freaking big deal. Let's look at some of the ways in which they can be affected.

Shock and fear

Your partner will very likely have been impacted by the initial cancer diagnosis. They too will have experienced the shock and fear that comes with the BAM-moment of hearing that you have cancer. Whilst they were not told that *they* had cancer, to hear that you, their partner and loved one, has cancer will have been decidedly shocking, scary and overwhelming. Just as you may have feared for your life at this point, so may your partner have feared for your life.

The emotional toll

There's a definite emotional toll to being the partner of someone going through cancer. Your partner will probably have provided you with emotional support throughout all the tests, scans, waiting for results and appointments at which you may have had difficult conversations about the extent of your cancer and your prognosis. Equally, it may also take an emotional toll on someone to see their partner suffer from the harsh side-effects of cancer treatment. The emotional toll of supporting a loved one through all of this cannot, quite honestly, be underestimated.

Disagreeing on decisions

Your partner will have most likely been involved in discussing and making difficult treatment decisions with you. Whilst ultimately all the treatment decisions were yours to make, most people turn to their partners to help with the decision-making process. And what if you disagreed on some of the decisions? What if there were difficult discussions over some of the decisions? This would have been hard for them.

Taking on extra responsibilities at home

Your partner may have had to take on more responsibilities at home: cooking, cleaning, child care, walking the dog, putting out the bins, tidying the house, doing the food shop and so on. Usually, these sorts of responsibilities are shared, but if one of the couple is regularly at hospital receiving treatment or feeling ill from the side-effects of treatment, the other one inevitably has to take on more. This can be overwhelming and it can be made all the more difficult when trying to juggle all the extra responsibilities with work and supporting you through treatment.

Being a primary caregiver

Your partner may have been your primary care-giver during your treatment. Taking on this role – on top of everything else – will have been hard work in terms of juggling everything that was going on.

Emotional needs

Your partner may not have had an outlet for his/her own emotional needs. Given what you've been going through, and the fact that they've been supporting you on an emotional level, it's unlikely that they will

159

have turned to you for emotional support. It's quite possible that they haven't sought any support for themselves as they support you and the rest of the family through this difficult time.

No time for themselves

With all the extra responsibilities and everything else that cancer brings to a family, your partner may have less – or no – time for their own interests or seeing their friends. A lack of their 'own time' can also be a contributing factor to increased stress.

Facing their mortality

Cancer can trigger anxiety in your partner: whilst you've faced your mortality square in the face, it's highly likely this has caused them to think about their own mortality. Addressing things like death and mortality can be very stressful.

The impact on your relationship with your partner

Not only are partners impacted on their own terms in the ways just described, let's not forget that when one of a couple is going through cancer it can be a really rather testing time for the relationship. Sadly, relationships can be impacted in a variety of ways, such as:

An emotional support imbalance

Cancer patients have emotional needs for which they turn to their partners: the need to be listened to, heard, understood and supported, 100 per cent. What if their partner can't provide that emotional support in the way the patient needs? And what about the partner's emotional needs – the patient can't take these on so where does the partner go for support? The usual ways in which a couple rely upon one another for – and in turn provide – emotional support can completely change during cancer leading to an emotional support imbalance.

Sexual intimacy

This will inevitably be impacted by one of the couple going through cancer treatment. And in the case of breast cancer treatment, sexual intimacy can be affected well after the end of treatment thanks to the side-effects of hormone therapy and an induced menopause. Sadly, comments such as this one, are very common, *'Being intimate has been hard at times due to my sickness, recovery from surgery and the impact of the menopause symptoms'.*

Resentment and frustration

Considering all the extra responsibilities and lack of emotional support, a partner may experience complicated feelings of resentment and frustration as they care for their loved one through treatment.

Changes in roles

Each partner has their own role in the relationship and within the family. However, when one partner is unable to fulfil their usual role, and the other has to step in, this can lead to a raft of issues. For example, the unwell partner might not be happy about their partner stepping into their role and they may try to control how this is done – which could be read by their partner as a lack of trust. On the other hand, the well partner might not step into their ill partner's role and this can lead to feelings of frustration. Essentially, the couple is seeing their partner in a new light, and they may not like what they see.

Changes in physical appearance

The physical side-effects of treatment can alter the appearance of someone: hair loss, weight changes, surgical scars and in the case of breast cancer, mastectomies, lumpectomies and reconstruction will all lead to physical changes. Sadly, some partners can struggle with the physical changes of their partner. Partners may have an underlying – almost subconscious – perception of what they want a woman to look like. In the case of breast cancer surgery, the physical changes can bring this perception to the fore, potentially creating an issue in the relationship.

Back to normal

As we looked at in Chapter 11, it's quite possible that after treatment your partner will assume that you're okay and that life will return to normal. It could be a genuine expectation on their part, or it could be a case of 'wishful-thinking'. Of course, a partner will just want everything to go back to normal once treatment is over. They've just been through a horrific time, and all they want is everything to go back to the way it used to be. It's common for people to (sometimes subconsciously) take the view that for an illness to be valid, it has to be visible: *you look ill so therefore you are ill and I will adapt my behaviour accordingly by helping out and supporting you.* When someone doesn't look ill, it's harder for people to accept that the person is ill: *you look better so you must be fine.* They don't see the invisible impact of cancer as it lingers on after treatment and this can result in someone not understanding the position of their partner or spouse. Sadly, comments like this are all too common, *'My relationship suffered as a result of me having had cancer. I became angry with my partner because I felt that as soon as I had been given the all clear he thought I should be 'over it'.*

Highlighting the cracks

Oh, and let's not forget that cancer can highlight pre-existing cracks in the relationship: things that had been going on before cancer but which had not been acknowledged or addressed. A couple can have plenty of stressors in their relationship – for example, aging parents, problems at work or existing psychological issues. Sometimes, a relationship just can't cope with all of the stress that it's put under and the addition of another stress factor – cancer – can be a wake-up call for the couple that their relationship is struggling.

What to do to help your partner and relationship

That's an awful lot for a partner to go through and an awful lot for a relationship to go through. All this naturally leads to the question, what can you do about the impact of your cancer diagnosis on your partner and relationship? Thankfully Barbara is here to help. Her advice is:

- Talk to your partner. Talk about the impact of your cancer on them, and on your relationship. Open communication may be difficult for some people but it can help to identify any issues that can then be worked on.
- Remember to be aware that there will be differences between the two of you and it's important to show respect for each other's views. Going through a traumatic life experience, like cancer in a relationship, can highlight issues and differences that might not have previously been there or were hidden under the surface of the relationship.

- Each of you might believe that you're right and so it's about finding an agreeable point in the middle that works for you both. This might make things uncomfortable for you, so think about how you make that discomfort bearable.
- Be patient with each other and with yourself. The way that you feel immediately after the end of treatment might (and it usually does) change over time.
- It's worth considering seeing a professional for couples therapy or family therapy if things feel particularly difficult.
- Many women who've had breast cancer find sexual intimacy difficult after treatment due to the impact of hormone therapy on their libido and due to pain caused by vaginal dryness arising from hormone therapy. It's important to talk to your spouse about what you're experiencing. There is some excellent specialist advice about this. Take a look at the Useful Resource section for some recommendations.

As a general note when it comes to the impact of your cancer upon your family, Barbara says that if you notice that you are blaming yourself or feeling guilty for what is happening to your partner and children, please stop. That is not a healthy or useful way for you to spend your limited energy. You might like to take a look at Chapter 16 which talks about coping with feelings of guilt.

Issues arising from your community

It's worth mentioning here that in some cultures – for example, some British Asian communities and some black communities within the U.K. – someone can face additional challenges both during and after a cancer diagnosis. Sometimes talking about cancer and its impact is a taboo subject; unhelpful myths about cancer can be prevalent within the community; someone who has – or has had – cancer can be stigmatised by members of their family or community; or cancer and its impact is just misunderstood by people within a community – and hence their family. Facing such challenges from your family, culture or community can add additional hurdles to those that you are already trying to overcome as you process what you've been through and try to move on from having had cancer.

This is a sensitive and complicated subject to cover, and it is beyond the remit of this book. However, I'm going to touch upon it briefly here because if you are in this situation, it's important to understand that you are not alone in what you are going through.

Let's take the example of Iyna, a British South Asian Muslim woman who was brought up within a traditional Muslim community here in the U.K. She was diagnosed with primary breast cancer at the age of 30. Speaking to her, seven years after her diagnosis, she told me that dealing with the aftermath of cancer has been incredibly challenging:

'I was brought up to understand that my individuality wasn't as important as my family and community: throughout my life, I haven't felt allowed to put myself first. So, when I finished my breast cancer treatment (which in itself was difficult because of my Muslim culture) and I was faced with all sorts of emotional issues about who am I and what my purpose is, it was really the first time in my life that I was actually thinking about me and putting myself first. I realised that I was my own person and I wanted to do things that make me happy. I wanted to progress my career, I wanted to live my life according to my plans, and I wanted to speak out about my breast cancer experience and help other British South Asian Women who were going through it. But it's been really hard and I feel alone. I feel guilty for wanting to live my life in this way. My family doesn't understand – I think they feel betrayed by me and that I'm being selfish. I don't want to upset my family – I want to be able to live my life in this way whilst also being a good, supportive daughter, sister and member of the community, but I'm not sure they can accept this'.

Iyna's experience is just one example. You may have faced something similar, or you may have a different experience of cultural issues impacting your recovery from cancer. And you may be feeling scared, shamed, guilty, burdened, confused, misunderstood and alone. But you are not alone. There are plenty of other people like you and whilst it might be difficult to do so, it can be helpful to seek out those who are experiencing similar challenges within your culture or community with whom you can share experiences and provide valuable support for one another.

There are currently a few – although sadly not many – cancer support groups in the U.K. dedicated to supporting people within these communities. Take, for example, the Black Women Rising movement founded by Leanne Pero. Leanne went through breast cancer as a black woman aged 30, six years ago. Leanne says:

'Faced with a myriad of challenging reactions to my diagnosis from my community in South East London, I went through treatment feeling utterly alone. It was after completing treatment that I realised that what I had experienced as a young black woman, wasn't unusual within my community and so I set up the Black Women Rising cancer support project to bring together women from black and Asian communities to provide support, education and help women who are facing cultural issues from within these communities'.

Looking for, and reaching out to, people for support can feel incredibly daunting. But just remember that there are lots of other people just like you who are also looking to reach out. Social media can be a great starting point from where to connect with other people who are experiencing similar issues and challenges to yourself. It's also worth speaking to your breast care nurse or other members of your medical team as they might be able to put you in touch with other people or may be able to point you in the direction of local support groups. Equally, you can get in touch with the national charities (their email addresses and support helplines are displayed on their websites) and ask if they are aware of any specific support groups for people in your situation. The key is to find people who are experiencing the same or similar challenges to you, and with whom you can share stories, advice and support one another.

Top tip

Don't blame yourself for the way in which your cancer has impacted your family.

Checklist

Here's a recap of the key points for you to take away from this chapter.

1 Do not blame yourself or feel guilty for the way that your cancer has impacted your family.
2 Sometimes it can help to involve other family members and good friends in ascertaining the impact of your cancer on your child.
3 Talk to your children about their feelings and respond appropriately. Don't ignore or deny what they are feeling.

4 Find the space and time to regularly talk to each child on a one-to-one basis.

5 The way in which you will talk to your child, and how you can reassure them, will depend on their age and emotional maturity.

6 Keep an open dialogue with your child's school about what is going on at home and how they are behaving at school.

7 Consider whether you should seek professional help for your child.

8 Adult children can also be impacted by your cancer, so it can be helpful to have an open conversation with them about how they are feeling.

9 Be aware that going through a traumatic life experience like cancer can highlight issues and differences that might not previously have been there or were hidden below the surface of the relationship.

10 Try to have open communication with your partner about the impact of your cancer on them and your relationship. But recognize that this might be difficult for some people.

11 Be patient with each other. The way that everyone feels immediately after the end of treatment can change over time.

12 Consider whether you and your partner would benefit from couples therapy or family therapy.

13 The good news is that sometimes cancer can also highlight the strengths of your partner and relationship so it's not all negative news.

14 Seek out others in your situation who will understand what you're going through and with whom you can each support one another.

Notes

Use this page to plan out how you could help your children and partner cope with your cancer diagnosis.

16

Guilt

The guilt of having had cancer and its impact on others

'Guilt is huge. Guilt for what happened to my family and all of the uncertainty and fear. Guilt for the worry my parents endured. Guilt at leaving my kids when I was in hospital. Guilt at not being able to properly look after my baby when I had surgery. Guilt even now. Guilt when the kids are annoying me because I shouldn't feel that way after cancer. Guilt when I hear of other women having a recurrence because even as I feel sympathy for them, a part of me thinks "it's not me today". Guilt that, on some days, I'm a nervous wreck and my husband has to put up with me'.

Natasha

As you will have come to understand by now, there is a bucket load of complex emotional issues to deal with at the end of cancer treatment. The next one to talk about is guilt. Cancer and guilt: it's a double act. Unfortunately, it's not a comedy double act but more of a dark, brooding, grip-your-heart-in-its-hands double act. It's a double act right from diagnosis all the way through treatment and it doesn't always go away when treatment ends. In fact, the feelings of guilt are sometimes at their peak after treatment.

The different ways in which guilt can be felt

Of course there are questions about how to deal with the guilt associated with having been through cancer, but let's start by exploring some of the guilty feelings that you might be experiencing at this stage so you can see how what you're feeling is totally normal and how you're experiencing similar feelings to many other people. There's a myriad of ways in which someone might feel guilt associated with their cancer but together with Anne Crooke (the Counsellor in psycho-oncology who has helped with insight and advice in one of the earlier chapters) we've picked out the most common ways in which someone may feel guilty after a cancer diagnosis.

Guilt about the impact of your cancer on your children

As parents, we're programmed to feel guilty about everything we do and don't do when it comes to our children. We feel guilty for not giving them enough of our attention; guilty for allowing them too much screen time; guilty for putting them in the after-school club and on and on and on. Almost everything we do and every decision we make is subconsciously measured against our inbuilt guilt-o-meter.

Now take a cancer diagnosis. It's highly likely that if you're a parent, your guilt-o-meter readings will have been off the scale ever since you received your diagnosis. I know they were for me, and when I talked to Kathryn as part of my research for this book, she told me:

> 'I feel an overwhelming guilt if I'm shut away in my room dealing with fatigue and anxiety, and I can hear my parents playing with my daughter'.

And Vicky explained:

> 'I feel guilty as a parent that my children have had to find out about cancer at such an early age'.

It's perfectly normal to have feelings of guilt surrounding your cancer and your children. You may have felt guilt about things such as:

- Causing your children to be scared and anxious about the fact that one of their parents has cancer: we associate cancer with the possibility of death so we inevitably assume that our children will also associate our diagnosis with the possibility of our death.
- Causing disruption to normal life: hospital appointments which impact upon the school run; the inability to have friends over or go to friends' houses; and holiday cancellations.
- Not being able to do as much with the children because of the side-effects, whether that's playing with younger children, taking the children out and about, or supporting older children who're going through important exams or other important life changes.
- Putting your child in a position where they have to see you at your worst as you deal with side-effects, fatigue and possibly hair loss.

Just a little note here, whilst this chapter will provide some insight and advice on how you deal with these feelings of guilt, it's worth revisiting Chapter 15 for advice on coping with the impact of your cancer upon your children.

Guilt about the impact of your cancer on your parents

Some of you reading this will have older parents who have supported you through your cancer diagnosis and treatment. It's common to feel guilt for putting parents through the emotional stress of their child having cancer. Again, given that we associate cancer with the possibility of death, we inevitably assume that our parents will also associate our diagnosis with the possibility of our death which will lead to stress, worry and anxiety for them. Take Vicky, for example, who simply said to me:

> 'I feel guilt towards my parents for causing them worry'.

Many of you will also have relied upon older parents for help and support throughout treatment: help with childcare, lifts to the hospital, company for hospital appointments and treatment; and general help at home. This can inevitably lead to feelings of guilt at requiring more from your parents than usual, taking up their time and putting them under physical stress.

Guilt about your partner

As we saw in the previous chapter, it's often a partner who bears the brunt when it comes to a cancer diagnosis. You could say that partners go through cancer without actually having it. They are around for all the stressful appointments; they see their loved one go through tough – sometimes harsh – treatment; and they stand by watching them grapple with a myriad of horrible side-effects. Partners have to step up at home, do more around the house and more of the child care, all the while supporting their loved one and usually working at the same time. And on top of all this, they have to deal with – often silently – the stress and worry about their loved one having cancer.

If you feel this way, then you're certainly not alone. Vicky explained to me:

'I feel guilt towards my husband that our lives have changed so much and that I've generally lost a bit of my shine. The induced menopause has had the expected effect on our personal life and I hate this'.

And Ruth told me:

'Guilt weighs heavily on me. I feel guilty on so many levels: that I've put my loved ones through this and that the first year of my relationship was taken from me'.

Whilst this chapter will provide insight and advice to help you deal with these feelings of guilt, it's worth revisiting Chapter 15 for advice on coping with the impact of cancer on your partner.

Survivor's guilt

Survivor's guilt is the guilt that someone feels for surviving cancer when so many people don't. It might be guilt about someone in particular – a friend or someone they met at the hospital – or it might just be a general feeling of guilt that they didn't die but many other people do die from the disease. It's certainly not unusual for someone to feel this way, and many of the women I interviewed for this book told me that they were experiencing survivor's guilt to some extent. Jo H told me:

'I also suffered with huge feelings of guilt, guilty because I had been so lucky but was getting in such a state yet there were people younger than me with much worse outcomes than mine'.

Guilt for all the help you've received and for being a burden

While you were going through cancer, the chances are that you'll have received plenty of help and support from friends, neighbours, family and even from people you hardly know. People will most likely have done all sorts of helpful things, like brought you meals for your freezer, taken the kids off your hands, done a food shop for you and taken you to and from hospital appointments. They've taken time out of their day to help you. And this is all so wonderful, amazing and appreciated. But when treatment is over and you don't need quite as much help, you might reflect on how everyone helped out and feel that you've been a burden to them:

'Due to my fatigue and pain, my parents often look after my three-year-old daughter for me. I feel guilty that my parents have to help me out so much and that I am such a burden to them'.

Kathryn

Guilt about doing the wrong things and increasing the risk of getting it again

Yet another example of guilt is the guilt that someone may feel about doing the wrong things and increasing the risk of getting cancer again. Plenty of people – including me – feel guilty about how they are not doing everything that they can possibly do to prevent the cancer from coming back. For example, they might feel guilty for not exercising as much as they've been told they should do to help prevent cancer; for being stressed at work when they've heard that stress can cause cancer; and they might have read that a particular diet can help prevent a return of their cancer and so if they don't follow this particular diet – or they don't follow it to the letter – they are increasing their risk of recurrence.

Such diets usually involve cutting out all sorts of things like sugar, dairy, meat and alcohol so eating a cupcake that your child made for Easter, having a glass of wine to celebrate a birthday or eating something containing dairy can lead to huge feelings of guilt. Rachel L said to me:

> 'I feel guilty that I haven't lost weight, that I sometimes eat sugar, that I don't move my body enough, that I'm not fit and if I get a recurrence, it will be all my fault. I've already put my family and friends through enough, I don't want to have to do it again'.

And Kathryn explained:

> 'Not being in control of my own body has led to my anxiety. I worry that there must be something that I can do to prevent a recurrence of cancer, so I research all sorts of supplements and diets – but all this does is to fuel the anxiety because if I end up eating something that I've read can increase cancer, I feel terrible guilt and I worry that I've just increased the chances of the cancer coming back'.

Why do people feel guilty?

There are so many things to feel guilty about when it comes to cancer. How on earth can you deal with all this guilt? Well, Anne suggests that to start with, it's helpful to understand *why* people feel guilt. This requires us to go back to basics and look at the meaning of guilt itself. Guilt is a feeling of responsibility or remorse for committing a wrong, whether real or imagined. It's actually a helpful emotion for life generally: if we feel that we've transgressed or acted in a way that has caused some harm, feeling guilt for this transgression or harm becomes helpful as it allows us to realize our actions have had a consequence that we regret and it encourages us to want to make it right. We can then apologize, make reparations and remember to not do the same thing again.

As you can see, guilt implies some agency on our part – it requires us to do something wrong whether deliberately or unwittingly. However, having cancer is not down to doing something wrong: there hasn't been any choice in getting cancer. Let's be clear, cancer is a random event down to cells working in a random way. So, unlike the true meaning of guilt, someone who has had cancer cannot use the guilt to make reparations, apologize or remind themselves not to do it again. Guilt is not serving its proper purpose here.

So why do people feel 'guilt' for having had cancer and for the impact this has had on others around them? It's a good question and one that is perhaps too extensive for the purpose of this book. So, we're going to look at the feelings of post-cancer guilt in one particular way. That is, the way that some people use 'guilt' to possibly mask other emotions: it's quite possible that describing an emotion as 'guilt' is an interpretation of how you're feeling bad about something. If you can go behind the 'guilt' and look at and process what you're actually feeling bad about, it might help you to move on from both feeling 'guilty' and whatever feelings are behind the guilt.

Yep, that all sounds a little complicated so let's take each of the examples of the way in which people often feel 'guilty' after cancer that were highlighted at the start of this chapter, and with Anne's help we can unpack these feelings:

Guilt about the impact of cancer on your children

According to Anne, the guilt that you feel towards your children could be partly to do with the expectations that you have of yourself as a parent. Everyone wants to be the best possible parent and part of being the best possible parent is protecting your child from distress and bad things happening to them. So, if bad things happen to your child, or your child suffers distress, you'll inevitably feel bad that you're not being the best possible parent.

However, in reality, bad things do happen in life and can happen to anyone. Take your cancer diagnosis for example. Cancer of a parent certainly falls within the definition of a bad thing happening to your child. Something bad has happened to your child which makes you feel like you are not living up to your expectations of being the best possible parent. And so it's natural to feel bad about this.

But let's look at what it means to be a good parent. Part of being a good parent is guiding your child through bad things and distressing experiences. It's about showing them how to build resilience and manage the pitfalls in life, equipping them with the skills and resources for managing whatever situation they find themselves in. It's about supporting them through these difficult situations by helping them find strategies.

So, if you can help your child to manage the experience of you having had cancer, then surely this is being a good parent and you don't need to feel bad, or 'guilty'. Remember that Chapter 15 provides some insight and advice for helping you deal with the impact of your cancer diagnosis on your family.

Guilt about the impact on your loved ones and about being a burden to them

It's perfectly normal to feel 'guilt' that your cancer has had an impact on those around you and 'guilt' for being a burden. There's no escaping the fact that your cancer will have impacted your partner, parents and close friends on a practical level as well as an emotional level. They will probably have had to take time out of their normal days to provide practical help such as childcare or driving you to the hospital. And emotionally, it's more than likely that they'll have been feeling worried, anxious and stressed throughout the whole process.

Let's take a closer look at all of this with Anne. First of all, she suggests that it's important to recognize that what they've been going through – whether the stress or the extra time they've been giving you – is not your fault. It's cancer's fault. And it's not your fault that you had cancer. Have another look at the definition of guilt and the purpose of guilt. You have not done anything wrong.

Now, let's look behind these feelings of 'guilt' to see if there are some other emotions and feelings that you can identify and then process. Have a look at this set of questions that Anne has put together:

- Do you feel bad because others have had to help you more than usual? Is this more about the feelings of vulnerability that cancer brings with it? Needing help from others is a constant reminder of being unwell.
- Have you felt frustrated at the change in your role from capable mother/wife/daughter to someone in need of help and support? Have you felt frustration at the changes to the balance of these relationships where you've needed these people more than before? Have you felt frustration at having to reset your expectations of yourself?

It can be hard to hold a positive image of yourself in the relationship (whether with your partner, parents or friends) and be unable to fulfil that role – your whole sense of self can change.

- Are you distressed that rather than being the carer, you've had to be cared for?
- Are you feeling sadness that you've been unable to reciprocate the help they've been giving to you?
- Are you sad that your partner, parents and close friends have had to make extra time for you, rather than doing nice things like, maybe going on holiday?
- Are you concerned by the stress that they've been under?
- Are you angry that cancer has not just impacted you, but those around you?

Anne says that if you can identify the emotions and feelings behind the guilt you feel towards your family and close friends, you can then take steps to process those emotions and feelings. Being able to name the emotions behind the guilt (such as anger, frustration, sadness, vulnerability and concern) is the first step to being able to process how you are feeling.

Back to the best friend exercise: imagine that your best friend is the one going through these emotions, what would you say to them? What would your kind and compassionate response be to them in this situation? It's also worth looking again at Chapter 15, which provides some insight and advice for helping you deal with the impact of your cancer diagnosis on your family.

Guilt about doing the wrong things and increasing the risk of getting cancer again

Anne acknowledges that after cancer it's natural to want to do things that help prevent cancer from returning and often this involves making lifestyle changes such as changing your diet, increasing your exercise activity, stopping smoking and reducing alcohol intake. This is all good. After all, doing all of these things will certainly benefit your health. However, she warns that it's really important to remember that it's all about balance. Without balance, there is a risk that you'll feel bad if you can't keep up these changes and this is what can lead to feelings of guilt in these situations.

Here's a typical example of the kind of situation that Anne regularly sees in her post-cancer patients. Take, someone – let's call her Abi – who has read that sugar can increase the risk of a cancer recurrence.[1] Abi has decided to completely cut out all sugar in her diet. But then her daughter comes home from school with a batch of cupcakes she made in food tech class and she asks Abi to try one. As a mother, Abi feels obligated to have one. Given the fact that these cupcakes were made with sugar, Abi feels terrible that she's just eaten sugar. She's convinced herself that by eating that cupcake, she's increased the chances of a cancer recurrence and she's feeling 'guilty'.

As you can see, explains Anne, behind Abi's 'guilt' are feelings associated with the fear of recurrence and the lack of control surrounding recurrence. The driver behind giving up sugar is wanting to be in control, in a situation where there is an element of uncertainty which can't be controlled. But cancer is random and whilst adopting a healthy lifestyle will reduce the risk of recurrence, it cannot be entirely eliminated and there will always be a risk of recurrence.

People continue to beat themselves up for slipping off their new healthy regimes. But – an Anne reminds us – it's all about balance and recognizing that the risk of recurrence cannot be taken away completely: trying to make healthy choices that contribute to lowering the risk of recurrence but not depriving yourself of everything pleasurable. Depriving yourself of everything pleasurable, such as a cupcake or a glass of wine, is like punishing yourself for having had cancer. It was bad enough going through what you've been through, so now that you've made it out the other side and you have a life to live, it's important to live it healthily and with enjoyment, without the enjoyment instilling a feeling of guilt. Balance and moderation are the key words here.

Survivor's guilt

Survivor's guilt is the guilt that someone feels for having survived cancer whilst others have not. With survivor's guilt there is certainly an element of guilt in the truest sense of the word, but there is also the possibility that the guilty feeling is masking something else. Anne suggests that it could be a front for feelings such as:

- Asking the *Why me?* question. Questioning why you've survived cancer, whilst others haven't, often leads to questioning why you got cancer in the first place. Chapter 6 covers this.

- A fear of recurrence. Seeing your worst-case scenario play out before your eyes, whereby someone else has been where you are, and then developed secondary cancer and died will naturally increase your fear of the cancer recurring or spreading and causing your death. Chapter 5 covers coping with the fear of recurrence.
- Vulnerability, uncertainty and feelings surrounding the fragility of life. Thinking about this sort of thing can often invoke a sense of your own mortality, which can lead to anxiety. Chapter 4 deals with coping with anxiety.

Advice for dealing with feelings of guilt

So, there you go. You can see, can't you, how feelings of 'guilt' can mask other emotions. This is all very well but the next – natural – question is how do you know whether your feelings of 'guilt' are masking such emotions and feelings? Thankfully, Anne's here to help us with this. Anne suggests that there are two main questions to ask yourself when you're experiencing feelings that you label as 'guilt':

1 Am I using 'guilt' to punish myself for what I perceive I've put myself and others through?

or

2 Does my 'guilt' mask some other emotions or feelings arising from having had cancer?

Let's look at the first question to start with. Anne suggests that given guilt is an unpleasant, uncomfortable feeling, it can be self-punishing to feel guilty. For someone who feels bad that their cancer has had an impact on those around them, it's easy to get stuck in the guilty feeling as a way of punishing yourself for some upset or damage that you perceive you've caused them. But, as Anne has explained, cancer is not your fault so you don't need to punish yourself. You've been through enough and now is the time to show yourself compassion and kindness. Would you punish someone else for going through cancer? Of course you wouldn't. So, give yourself a break and stop punishing yourself for having been through something that was totally out of your control.

Now taking the second – more difficult – question. As explained in the preceding sections of this chapter, it's worth looking at your feelings of guilt to see whether there are other emotions behind this. Anne suggests that to do this, you could try to sit with the feelings and think about what else is going on. It can be really rather uncomfortable to do this and you might prefer not to do this on your own but with a trained professional or a good friend. However you decide to do it, here are some questions that you could ask yourself:

- Are you feeling 'guilty' about something that is beyond your control?
- Is that a kind, fair and compassionate way to talk to yourself? Would you see it the same way if it was a friend describing the situation to you?
- Is the 'guilt' you're feeling masking a feeling that seems harder to be with?

It can be helpful to write down your thoughts to help work out what emotions and feelings are going on. Why not grab yourself a cup of coffee and a pen, then start thinking about your answers to these questions using the notes page at the end of this chapter. The answers to these questions should help you work out what you're dealing with. The next step is to then process those feelings and emotions. You might want to do this by re-reading the chapters in this book that deal with the relevant feelings and emotions. Or, if you're struggling with this exercise and can't seem to move beyond the 'guilt' it might be sensible to seek professional help from, for example, a psychologist or counsellor.

Top tip

Imagine that your best friend comes to you and tells you that they feel guilt for exactly the reason that you're currently feeling guilty. Your best friend is, in fact, going through exactly what you're currently going through. What would you say to your friend about why they feel this way and how would you treat your friend?

Checklist

Here's a recap of the key points for you to take away from this chapter.

1 Be aware that feeling guilty can keep you stuck and prevent you from addressing the emotions behind the guilt and thus becoming more at ease with these feelings.

2 Feelings of guilt can continue for some time. And sometimes, it can feel easier to remain stuck in a nebulous feeling of guilt rather than try to address what's behind it. But it's important to do this.

3 Feeling guilty about something often leads to you feeling stuck in this bad feeling, so by reframing it to look at what is going on behind the 'guilt' can help you deal with some uncomfortable feelings and lessen some of the stress you might be putting on yourself.

Notes

Use this page to explore the emotions and feelings behind your guilt

17

The new normal

Coming to terms with the fact that life doesn't necessarily return to normal

'While going through treatment, you have to believe that life will go back to normal: this is what drives you to get to the end of treatment. But when you get to the end of treatment you realize that there is no 'normal'. Life is always going to be different'.

Gabi

As you got closer to the end of your cancer treatment, you may have had an expectation that life would return to the way it was before cancer: to normal days doing normal everyday things like going to normal work with normal people; doing normal things with friends; exercising normally; and generally having a normal life again. Furthermore, you may have been expecting and hoping that you would return to the person you were before cancer: back to the normal person in your head. In other words, that everything would go back to normal.

These thoughts will most likely have driven you to put one foot in front of the other for the entire period of treatment, whether that was a few months or years. It will have been a great motivator knowing that, if you just get through the next step of treatment, you'd be a little bit closer to getting back to normal you and normal life. In fact, it didn't even cross my mind that when I finished my treatment, my life would be anything but the way it had been before I'd had cancer.

But as you have come to understand, post-cancer life can be very different to life before cancer and you can feel like a different person to whom you were before your diagnosis. Allie Morgan – the Confidence Coach who has helped with some of the earlier chapters – says:

'It's worth understanding that when someone goes through a traumatic life event, such as cancer, it is perfectly normal to come out the other end as a different person. The extent of the difference will of course differ from person to person, but everyone will come out different in some ways'.

Yes, the extent to which life feels different post-treatment, differs from person to person and I like to think of it like a scale. Remember how I talked about this scale all the way back in Chapter 1? At one end of the scale are those – few – people for whom very little changes and who can, on the whole, return to the way they lived their lives before cancer. At the other end of the scale are those people for whom returning to anything resembling pre-cancer life feels out of reach. And then there is everyone else who falls somewhere within these two extremes. This is where the majority of people fall and for these people, some things will go back to normal but other things in their life might feel different. This is probably where you fall on the scale (after all it's the reason you're reading this book).

I started this book – back in Chapter 1 – by listing some of the ways in which you might feel physically, mentally and emotionally different now compared to the way you felt before you had cancer. And then over the course of the book – with help from the wonderful women who've talked to me about their experiences and the amazing experts who've provided their professional advice and insight – I've shown you that what you're feeling is normal, that you're not alone in how you're feeling and how you can start to cope with these new feelings. Even if you're only experiencing a couple of these feelings, they are probably new feelings that you've only had since cancer.

But it's not just these physical, mental and emotional changes that you might be experiencing: there are other ways in which your life can feel different now. So much can change once you've been diagnosed with cancer, that the way you think about life can be very different after having cancer. Going through cancer treatment and embarking upon your recovery can slow you down, and this sometimes provides opportunities for contemplation, deliberation, pondering and reflections about things such as:

- The realization that you could possibly die: it's likely that you'll have thought about your mortality and seriously wondered whether you'll survive.
- The important things in life: you may have reprioritized the things that are important to you and discovered that some of these were missing from your pre-cancer life.

- Your identity: you may feel as if your identity has changed – whether professionally or personally.
- Relationships and friendships: having seen the true sides of your friends during your treatment, you may have re-evaluated who you want in your life going forward.
- The fragility of life: that it's not a given that you'll live until a ripe old age of ninety but that people can die at any age and at any stage of their life.
- Your plans and goals: the life plan that you had before your diagnosis may have been severely altered by your cancer diagnosis.
- The sustainability of the way in which you were living your life: maybe taking a step back and looking at your pre-cancer life has shown you that you were doing too much, had too much on your plate and that it just wasn't a healthy way of living.
- Work and your career: perhaps a break from work has made you realize that you no longer want to follow that career path and you want to do something else.
- The bigger picture: you may have come to realize that there's more to life than your little bubble.
- Your values: maybe you lost sight of the things that are important to you while living your pre-cancer life and you've re-evaluated what values are important now.
- Your purpose in life: perhaps your perception of the world and how you fit into it has changed.
- Bad things don't always happen to other people: you may have come to understand that bad things can happen to anyone.
- Gratitude and appreciation: perhaps you're grateful for, and you have an appreciation for, so much more than before cancer.
- Mortality: you may have come to the realization that death can be entirely random, unfair and possibly just around the corner

Given the ways in which your thinking/feeling/realizing/understanding may have changed – in addition to the emotional, mental and physical changes that you might be experiencing – the chances are that as you sit here reading this chapter, you're feeling like a different person to the person who was sitting in the consultant's office one minute before you were told you had cancer.

And this is where the phrase 'new normal' comes in. It's a phrase that's used to describe how you're feeling now: how you're feeling physically, mentally and emotionally and how you're now thinking/feeling/realizing/understanding. I mentioned this phrase very briefly in Chapters 1 and 3 but you may have heard this phrase from people in your support networks, friends who may have been through cancer themselves, on online forums, or on social media. I know that since the world has been through Covid lockdowns we have probably all heard this phrase, but until I reached the end of my treatment back in pre-Covid days, I'd never heard of this concept.

It's a phrase that can instil feelings of uncertainty, confusion, disorientation and even fear because at the end of the day all that most of us want to do once cancer treatment is over, is to go back to our old, familiar lives. We want to go back to what is normal for us. And the thought that this might not be possible, but that you may have to adapt to a new way of life – a new normal – can be really rather frightening.

It's frightening because we humans are creatures of habit: we like normality and we don't particularly like change. So, getting to where you are now, and realizing that contrary to what you've been expecting, you're not going to go back to normal, can be really scary. It's perfectly possible that you're feeling overwhelmed by the thought of moving forward with your life – especially given the changes.

But you can't move on by forgetting or ignoring the fact that you had cancer: it's such a life-changing event. And you can't forget or ignore the way that cancer has made you think about life. So, when it feels impossible to return to normal – back to life as you knew it and back to a familiar you – how can you move forward? Yes, it's a time to be excited about getting on with your life, but how do you move on when so much has changed? There are two key issues to consider here: how can you find your new normal and how can you adapt to – and navigate – this new normal?

Before we look at these questions, Dr Jane Clark (the wonderful Consultant Clinical Psychologist who has provided so much support over the course of this book) has some reassuring words:

'Consider this … we all live according to the assumptions that we hold about life – it's our map of the world as we understand it. Before you had cancer you will have held certain assumptions about your life. You might have expected to live to a good old age and you would have lived your life making plans for the near and distant future based on that assumption.

The chances are that having been through cancer though, you'll now think differently. Having a traumatic diagnosis of cancer can shatter those assumptions and tear apart your map of the world and your understanding of how life works. You probably realize now that there are no certainties to living a long life, but things can happen to anyone and nobody has a guarantee of living to old age. This can feel destabilizing and like a fundamental change in your view of the world.

So, given that your old map of the world has been torn apart, you have to start again. You have to rebuild a new map: one that works in this new post-cancer reality of yours. And this isn't an easy process – it's a massive psychological shift to have to build a new map based on new assumptions. You'll be considering things like adapting to living with uncertainty, reviewing your purpose, grieving things you have lost, and considering changes to your priorities. And this can be really hard to do, particularly at a time when you might generally have low reserves.

Be kind to yourself as you're rebuilding your understanding of the way that life works. And give your mind a chance. After all, your mind has been living in accordance with one map for the entirety of your life and it's not going to be easy to start a new map, especially one based on so much uncertainty'.

It's all very well reading how the impact of cancer can change a person and the way they live and think, but in reality, it may not feel so black and white for you right now. You might still be processing some of the mental and emotional issues and whilst you may have noticed a change in the way you're thinking, you may not have given those thoughts the space and time to develop. It's a hell of a lot to take on board. If you're ready to consider this, then read on. But equally, if you think you need a little more time to process some of the things going on with you right now, just come back to this when you're ready.

For those of you ready to address this concept of the 'new normal', we're going to look at these two main issues with Allie:

- How can you find your new normal?
- How can you adapt to – and navigate – this new normal?

How can you find your new normal?

Turning to the first issue – finding your new normal – Allie recognizes that it can be hard to adapt when you're caught between wanting to go back to the comfortable old you, feeling different to the old you and not knowing how to find the new you. She says:

> 'It's perfectly natural to try to fit yourself into your old life, but cancer changes you in such a dramatic way that often it's just not possible to slot back into the old you and your old life. You have all this other experience behind you now, so you have to carve out a new path and work out what is best for you right now and going forward'.

Her advice is to start by thinking of this stage as starting a whole new era of your life; a rebirth after cancer. Acknowledge that you're not the same person as before cancer so don't try to fit back into your pre-cancer life. Don't worry – this doesn't mean that none of the old you remains, it's more a case that the whole picture is different because it's made up of newer parts as well as some of the old parts of you. The extent of the 'old you' that remains will differ from person to person and it's all a question of getting to know what has changed for *you*.

How can you adapt to – and navigate – this new normal?

So, the next step is to work out how you're different to the old you: what has changed? What's new? What hasn't changed? Allie's advice is to – for a brief moment – think about the person who sat in the chair seconds before they were told they had cancer. That was the old you. You don't need to worry about that person any more – they are in the past; you are now in the present and it's the present and the future that are important. It might help to say goodbye to that person, by perhaps writing them a letter.

However you think about the pre-cancer you, however you say good-bye to that person, now is the time to get to know the new version of yourself. You might be wondering how, exactly, you can get to know the new you. Well, this is the interesting part. It's not a quick process; it won't happen overnight and it can take some time. So, prepare yourself for the long game.

Allie suggests that you can start by thinking about how you would get to know a new friend or a prospective partner. You'd get to know them slowly, over a period of time. So, do the same with yourself. Ask yourself questions. Listen to your answers. Explore your feelings. Question your priorities. Probe your thoughts. Examine your values. This is where you need some time and space to process your thoughts. As part of this process, it might help to:

- Take yourself on some solo dates to a coffee shop with a notebook.
- Go for some long walks by yourself.
- Treat yourself to some selfcare evenings with long hot baths, soothing music and time to relax and think.
- Try meditation and mindfulness.
- Start writing and journalling.

Some of the things that you can ask yourself are:

- What has changed?
- How are you different?
- What are your priorities?
- How has your perspective changed on the things in your life?
- What do you want from your life?
- What are you appreciative of?
- What are you grateful for?
- What have you learnt by going through cancer?
- What is important to you?
- If you could change one thing about your life after cancer, what would it be and why?
- On a scale of 1–10, how satisfied do you feel in your career right now?
- What is your no. 1 goal for the next year?

As you'll see from all the other chapters in the book, your mind will be very busy at the moment coping with lots of stress, anxiety and scary thoughts. It's important to look beyond these when you're trying to get to know the new version of you.

Allie suggests that you look at the concrete evidence before you and don't focus on things that you can't control like, *What if my friends don't like the new me?* or *What if I can't do my job now?* Thoughts such as these are not supported by fact. You need to think about the facts. If you find that your mind is running away from you and you're worrying about what your new normal will look like (for example, *What if I'm made redundant?* or *What if I don't fit back in my old social circle?*) try writing a list of things based upon fact. For example:

- I've finished my cancer treatment.
- There is no cancer in me at the moment.
- I have a follow-up appointment booked for two months' time.
- I'm going back to work in one month and I'm going to phase myself back into work slowly.
- I know that my job is important to me and I'm grateful to have the opportunity to go back to work.
- I'm walking every day and I'm going to increase the distance that I'm walking every week.
- My friends have been incredibly supportive and I know who my true friends are.
- My family have been by my side throughout the cancer ordeal and I am so grateful for them.
- I'm incredibly grateful for …
- I appreciate …
- I love …

And all the while you're trying to get to know the new you and how your new normal life will look, don't be afraid to ask for help. If you're worried about the return to work, ask your employer to adapt the return so that it's not a big adjustment for you. If you're concerned about how your wider family will react to you, or how you'll fit back into social circles, talk to your family and friends about how you're feeling.

It's important to note that in adapting to your new normal, you don't need to make major changes. You don't need to run a marathon, write a book, start a charity or do something that you've seen other people doing on social media. You need to do what is right for you.

And it's important to recognize that the chances are that not everything about you or your life will change. The concept of a new normal might suggest that nothing will be the same as before you had cancer, but in reality, that's not the case. Let's go back to the scale again. Yes, there are some people at one end of the scale where everything will change: those who find that there is absolutely no 'back to normal' and instead they find a completely new way of living their life. These people want to use this time for change: they may find a new purpose; they may find growth opportunities; they may find enlightenment. But this is one end of the scale and most people fall in the middle where there are some changes, but also many aspects of pre-cancer life remain. It's a mix of new and old normal. And navigating a new normal will be different for everyone. For some people, there will be just a few changes while other people will make more.

Finally, remember that in life, nothing stays the same for ever. Normality isn't static, it's fluid. It will change over time. What's new for you now, will cease to be new in time, and something else will become new for you.

> **Top tip**
> Be kind to yourself as you're rebuilding your understanding of the way that life works and how you fit into it: it's a huge step to take.

Before leaving this chapter, I just want to tell you that you are not the only person feeling overwhelmed, confused, angry, or sad about the realization that life doesn't always go back to the way it was before cancer came knocking at your door. While interviewing all the wonderful women for this book, every one of them had something to say about the concept of the new normal and I'd like to share some of these with you...

'I'm definitely a different person to the one I was before cancer. I feel like I've been through a number of stages of transformation during treatment. I've had to go through a bit of a grieving process about losing the old me but I'm now embracing the new me I can't go back to my old life or the old me because I've gone through something that has evolved'.

Carly

'I'm determined not to be defined by cancer. I don't want to be "Gabi who had cancer". I want cancer to just be one episode in my life – an episode that had an impact on me, but which doesn't dictate the rest of my life. I'm struggling to get to that place. I thought that when you finished treatment, you'd click back into place and pick up where you left off. But it's not that straightforward'.

Gabi

'At the end of treatment, I was expecting to go back to normal but I didn't feel normal. I wanted to go back to who I was before cancer but I was very aware that I wasn't the same – I'd been forever changed by what had happened to me'.

Emily

'I thought that after my reconstruction surgery I would be able to just get back to normal as if I'd never been diagnosed with breast cancer. But then it hit me – this wasn't going to happen. I realized that I was never going to get my pre-cancer life back and instead I would have to learn to accept this new version of my life'.

Amy

'Life is complex post-treatment because there is everyday life and there is post-cancer life. I don't feel like me – I don't look like me and I know that I'm not me on a mental level'.

Molly

Checklist

Here's a recap of the key points for you to take away from this chapter.

1   There's no obligation to go back to the way you were before cancer, and there's no obligation to use cancer as a reason for changing yourself or your life. Do what feels right and natural for you. Don't force it, just go with what naturally happens.
2   It can be helpful to recognize and acknowledge that you are not exactly the same person as you were before you had cancer.
3   You might find it helps to say goodbye to the pre-cancer version of you, perhaps by writing a letter to that person
4   Get to know the new you. Writing and journalling can help, and you can ask yourself questions about your priorities, your values and your goals. The Toolkit at the back of the book provides some writing prompts to help you with this.
5   As you're getting to know the new version of you, focus on things based on fact and avoid thinking about the 'what ifs'.
6   Go on a 'moving forward' course – lots of hospitals, support centres and charities run these and they are aimed at helping you move on from cancer treatment by looking at the challenges that people in your position are facing, and working through them in an interactive setting.
7   Be patient with yourself and set reasonable expectations of how you'll adapt to your new normal.

Notes

Use this page to make notes on how and what you are thinking now in order to start to process your new normal.

18

Reflecting on life's priorities

Going through a traumatic life experience can cause you to re-evaluate and reprioritize

'I don't recognize the person I was before cancer. So many of my feelings and thoughts have changed'.

Nina

As you will have seen in the previous chapter, given what you've been through, it's often impossible to return to being exactly the same person you were before you had cancer, with the same beliefs, values and understanding of the world you live in. Part of moving forward after cancer can – for a lot of people although not everyone – involve creating a new normal. And part of creating a new normal can involve getting to know yourself by – as Allie suggested – questioning your priorities, probing your thoughts and examining your values. But it's not just a question of getting to know the new you, it's also understanding how you now look at life and the world generally.

Everyone is different when it comes to reflecting on life's priorities, resetting expectations and readjusting values. Some people may experience changes so slight that they hardly notice a change, whilst others may experience a much deeper shift. And some people might not even give this sort of thing any thought as they slot back into their pre-cancer way of thinking. There's no right or wrong way – it's all very personal. And equally, there's no pressure on you to have a change in mindset or even give this any thought.

For those of you who do reflect and undertake some introspective exploration, you might be interested to know that it's actually a natural way to move on from the traumatic experience that you've been through. It's not thanking cancer, or being grateful for having had cancer. You can't take away what you've been through and you can't forget it ever happened: it's part of you and always will be. As such, it'll naturally play a part in the way you look at your life and at the world in general, and it can change the way you view, value and think about certain things.

In fact, there's a term for this idea of personal growth after a traumatic event: it's called 'post-traumatic growth'.[1] Research has shown that people often reach a point after a traumatic event, when they have a new perspective on life. Some may call it a reawakening, some may refer to it as searching for meaning in life, and others may just realize what is, and isn't, important to them.

Research has also suggested that in order to reach post-traumatic growth, you might need to first process the traumatic event that you've been through. That is to say, rather than burying the difficult feelings inside you, you need to work through them. And post-traumatic growth doesn't happen overnight. It's a gradual process and constantly evolving.

Post-traumatic growth doesn't take the place of difficult emotions and feelings, it happens alongside them. You might still feel anxious or worry about cancer coming back, but your brain isn't consumed by fear. There is space for your brain to also have new feelings of appreciation and gratitude and to make re-evaluations and reprioritizations. It gives you room inside to grow, rather than always focusing on the fear and anxiety.

I've spent the past five years coming to terms with being diagnosed with cancer, and following the first of those five years when I went through treatment, I spent the past four years adapting – sometimes reluctantly – to my new normal. In doing so, I've used many of the exercises described in this book, and I've utilized many of the tools in the Toolkit. Over the course of the past four years, among other things, I've been processing anxiety and the fear of recurrence; coming to terms with the losses I experienced as a result of cancer; re-evaluating my purpose; adapting to the side-effects from hormone therapy; relearning to trust my body; rebuilding my confidence; and trying to answer 'why me?'. And alongside all of this, I've noticed that many of my values, goals, ideologies and views on life have changed and developed. I didn't go looking for these changes, but rather I've just come to understand them. I'd like to share some of my reflections, musings and observations with you...

Life isn't a race or a competition

'Slow down' has become a daily mantra for me and I'm actually fairly good at complying now. I wasn't very good at this before cancer. At the time of my diagnosis, I was multi-tasking motherhood/work/life and my life was busy, chaotic and somewhat crazy. Not only was day-to-day life a constant race, I was also rushing through my life: career, marriage, home, kids, family life and so on. Rushing from one thing to the next like it was a race to get to the next stage in life and a competition to get there in the most perfect way. I was desperate to get the 'look at my perfect life' medal. But there is no such medal and actually I now believe that we'll make personal wins if we slow down and savour every moment of our life as it happens.

We need to take the time to treasure every minute we have with our loved ones and make unforgettable memories with them. Life is happening now and we need to be present in the moment to appreciate it, not constantly looking ahead, planning and waiting for what tomorrow might bring. Because if we don't live in the moment while it's here, this moment will be gone. And before we know it, many moments will have gone without us really paying attention and we'll be asking ourselves, *Where did the time go?*

I talked to Cathy and Vicky about this and they both feel the same. Cathy explained to me:

'Life is very different now to before cancer. I am more mindful; I go through life at a slower pace and I am much more content to be at home. Cancer has turned down the adrenaline-fuelled life I was leading and I'm really happy. I cherish time with my family; I'm working less; I'm learning to take more time for me; I'm learning more about my health and taking action to keep healthy; I'm learning to relax; and I'm happy doing nothing and not feeling I have to be constantly busy'.

And Vicky told me:

'If I wake up on a beautiful day, I feel like I need to be out in that sunshine, I need to make those memories with my girls'.

Always be true to yourself

Authenticity and integrity are highly underrated. We often put on an exterior version of ourselves in order to fit in or conform to situations in life. We might do this subconsciously, or maybe at times we do it consciously. But the point is that we're not really showing our true selves to others.

We may wear certain outfits to go and pick the kids up from school because we think we'll only be accepted by the other mums if we look the part. We may put on a false air of confidence at work in order to be heard among the alphas in the team meetings. We may join in the gossip on a girls' night out because we want to fit in. By doing this, maybe we're subconsciously telling ourselves that our true versions are not good enough for other people. And so, often, this will lead us to feel unhappy about ourselves. Wouldn't it feel more comfortable, happier, liberating, if we showed our true authentic selves?

Both Carly and Nina also feel this way. Carly said to me:

'There's been an evolution during and after treatment, to me accepting the new me and connecting with the soul as opposed to what I place my material values on. I prefer the me now to how I used to be – I had a lot more self–loathing'.

And Nina explained:

'I had to let some friends go as they weren't on the same path as me. Thinking that I might die is a big thing to think about and inevitably it changed me. But the people around me hadn't changed and weren't in the same place as me'.

You can't pour from an empty cup

This is another favourite mantra of mine and I remind myself of this on a daily basis. We rush through life often putting ourselves at the bottom of the to-do list (that is if we even make it onto the to-do list in the first place). We run around putting the kids and partners – if we have them – work, home, friends and even pets before ourselves. And then we end up going to bed not having given ourselves a minute of attention throughout the day. We're too tired to sleep and we feel guilty about everything we haven't done for everyone else. This is not good. We keep on going until something breaks us, but surely, it's better to not get to the point of being broken in the first place.

We need to look after ourselves first and foremost. And we need to do this so that we can not only give ourselves to all the other things/people/ situations that are wanting/needing a part of us, but more importantly so that we feel good and enjoy this life we've been given. We need to regularly practise self-care, top up our reserves when they are low and recognize when things need to take a break. And we need to do all of this without feeling guilty.

Melissa agrees and she told me:

'Something has changed in me now, for the better. I feel like I've woken up! For a very long time I just put everyone before me. I was trying to be perfect: have the perfect home and life. It was exhausting. I really sweated the small stuff. I was a rushing woman, trying to be everything to everyone. Even when I thought I was being kind to myself it was never time I would give myself, but I'd treat myself to something like a new pair of boots. But now I know the importance of putting myself near the top of the list and doing the things that I want to do'.

And Jo H described her situation:

'My priorities have changed in the sense that I now put myself first sometimes. For so long it was always about what the kids wanted or needed but I realized it was fine to put my wants and needs first for a change'.

Letting go of control

Whilst we all have an element of control over our own lives, I now realize that it's deceptive to think that we have ultimate control of our lives. That if we do the right things, like eating healthily, exercising, and taking care of our bodies, and don't do the wrong things like smoking and drinking too much alcohol, then we'll live long healthy lives. We may think that we are in control but in reality, we're not. We're not in control of our destinies, but rather there is an element of randomness to life. We're not travelling along a defined road, but along one with bumps and forks and detours and diversions and dead-ends. At the end of the day, nobody knows where they'll end up.

The chances are you're doing the best you can

Whether it's being a parent, doing your job, running a business, looking after an elderly family member or being a good sibling or friend, you're probably doing the best you can. But we're often our own harshest critics and the chances are we all experience the 3 a.m. guilts at some point: *I can't be in two places at once and pick up the kids from school and take mum to the hospital – I am not a good enough mother or daughter; I had such a busy day that I forgot to text my friend to wish her happy birthday – I am such a terrible friend; I didn't call my brother to check how he got on at his job interview – I am such a terrible sister.*

But life is busy – often too busy – and things will happen that make us question if we're doing a good enough job. But we are! We're doing our best and that is all that we should expect from ourselves. Nina agrees. She told me:

> 'I used to work hard and have to travel all the time – my priorities have shifted and work is not the most important thing to me now: I just want to be present for my daughter'.

People are not talking about you behind your back

People are not talking about you behind your back and in any event, it doesn't matter what people think about you. It matters what you think about yourself. This goes back to my point about authenticity and integrity. If we can be comfortable in ourselves, then we will have less reason to fear what other people think about us. We mustn't value our self-worth by reference to what we think others think of us. It's what each of us thinks of ourselves that matters. Take Kathryn for example, who said to me:

> 'I feel different to the person I was before I had cancer. I'm less worried about what people think'.

We are not defined by our trauma

Going through a traumatic experience can take over life for a while. We end up living it, sleeping it, breathing it. Everything revolves around this traumatic experience. But then things settle down, life changes course and we can tentatively move forward. However, our trauma will often stay with us, even though to the outside world we've moved on. Of course it will – it was huge! But remember that the trauma doesn't define us. We are not just the trauma. We're made up from lots of parts: mother, daughter, sister, wife, friend, writer, dog-lover, cyclist, painter, singer, runner, hiker, volunteer, gardener, telly-watcher, reader, cook, whatever – everything and anything – it is we do. Factor in all our characteristics: quiet/loud, confident/shy, organized/disorganized, introverted/extroverted... our trauma is only a small part of us. It's not the whole of us and nor is it the biggest part.

It's okay to be sensitive and vulnerable

Life often instils in us an understanding that being sensitive and vulnerable is a sign of weakness: don't cry in front of people, put on a brave face, keep a stiff upper lip. You know the drill. It's also instilled in girls from a young age that in order to compete in a man's world we need to show the world that we are strong, self-assured, courageous women and we get to be those women by pushing down our sensitivities and vulnerability. By virtue of this, we come to believe that sensitivity and vulnerability are weaknesses that should be hidden. But perhaps it's actually a sign of strength to show these sides of our personality, rather than hide them.

Allowing ourselves to stop and acknowledge where we feel sensitive or vulnerable, allows us to seek help in dealing with these emotions and feelings, thus improving our emotional and mental health. In turn, this fosters greater resilience; an increase in emotional awareness; and improves our connection to those around us. Furthermore, it allows us to be comfortable with our authentic selves, and didn't I just tell you how important it is to be true to yourself rather than trying to be what you think other people want you to be?

I talked to Juliet about this and she explained to me:

'Seeing a counsellor has been a life changing experience for me. It's helped me understand myself, my behaviour, the way I think and how the way I think relates back to past experiences. I see counselling as a brave thing to do: it's not a sign of weakness but rather it's a sign of strength because you recognize that you can't help yourself and that you need help'.

Reading the accounts of people going through trauma, be it cancer, grief, divorce, depression or any other traumatic life event, will show you strong people putting their vulnerabilities out there for all to see, rather than shamefully hiding them away and putting on a brave face.

We all possess an inner strength of which we were previously unaware

Most of us are not especially brave, or inspiring, or special. We're just regular people going about our regular lives. However, I firmly believe that deep down, all of us possess an inner strength of which we are completely unaware until the time comes when this inner strength is required – whether that's a cancer diagnosis, the death of a loved one, a tricky divorce or some other traumatic life event. We just dig deep and draw out this special reserve of strength that is sitting in us, waiting for the time when we really need it. And everyone has this within them.

This issue of strength came up during many – if not all – of the interviews that I carried out for this book. Everyone agreed that just because we've been through cancer, we're not brave or inspiring, but there's something within everyone that can be tapped into when needed. For example, Carly told me:

'Being able to embrace the new you, shows a strength that we didn't know was there, and this shows that not everything that cancer gives us is bad. Cancer has been a huge experience which opens our eyes to our own mortality – the things you go through with cancer make you face things you would never normally face'.

And Molly simply said to me:

'I've realized how resilient I am'.

Nothing stays the same forever

Everything in life is in a state of impermanence. Back in Chapter 1 I introduced you to the Buddhist notion of Anicca: that all things and experiences are inconstant, unsteady, and constantly changing. Someone once told me this years ago at a point when I really needed to hear it and it's stayed with me ever since. And it's true. Whatever is going on today, will change over time and things won't be the same in maybe a week, a month or a number of years. It applies to everything in life: friendships, jobs, health, emotions. So, if something isn't going quite right for you at a particular moment remember Anicca and patiently wait for things to change. And equally, if things are going well and everything is great, remember Anicca – savour this time, make the most of it and enjoy it.

Life is about family and good, true friends

Life is about spending quality time with those we love and whom love us back. Life is about doing things and being with people who make us happy. Life is about being with people who push us forward and don't hold us back. It's about having people in our lives who support us, applaud us and make us feel good about ourselves. Not people who are jealous of our achievements, put us down and make us feel bad about ourselves. If ever there's an opportunity in life to re-evaluate who we want to have in our lives, it's now.

We all want to feel good and that is fine

At the end of the day, we all want to feel good. We want to be happy, feel content and occasionally experience joy. It's what we humans crave and everything we do in life comes down to this. It's just that sometimes, life can get in the way and we lose sight of the simplicity of this need: we often go a step further, perhaps we get greedy or perhaps we mistake other things for happiness. Things like material wealth, the number of Instagram followers, the designer labels in the wardrobe, being popular, reaching the top of the career ladder, a beautiful home – the list is endless. Yes, much of this will provide some form of pleasure, but sometimes it's at an emotional, mental or material cost to ourselves and/or those around us.

In fact, it can take a very bad experience – like cancer – to really understand that ultimately, everything circles back round to this need to feel good. Indeed, it's what this entire book has been about: processing and dealing with all the physical, emotional and mental obstacles to feeling good. Furthermore, it can take a very bad experience to remind ourselves that the process of reaching a good place is actually less complex than perhaps we'd been conditioned to believe in our pre-cancer days.

We can slow down, take stock and think about what makes us feel good and brings us happiness. We might realize that we don't need to race through life trying to accomplish hundreds of self-imposed goals, but that taking the slower, more mindful lane makes us happier. We might recognize that we've been putting on a pretence to the world but actually we'd be happier showing our true, authentic selves. We might want to purge our lives of toxicity: ditching the toxic people and situations in our lives. We might want to embrace new interests or rediscover old forgotten ones: having the confidence to take steps to bring such things into our lives. We might want to reset our boundaries: reminding ourselves of what is important to us. We might want to live a simpler, calmer life. We might want to spend more time with our families; choose the path with less conflict; practise more self-care or embrace our sensitivities and vulnerabilities. How we each get to our good place is up to each of us.

Life is too short to not feel good, find happiness or seek out moments of joy. So, to bring this book to a close, I'd like to share some reflections from a few of the wonderful women whom I interviewed for this book.

'Since cancer, I've learnt the importance of setting boundaries. It's so important to set our boundaries and not try to please everyone all the time. The only person who can give us inner peace is ourself and not the people or things around us. People and things add extra value to our lives but true happiness and joy is all down to me. My true happiness is being here, being with my daughter and being able to do the simplest things as going for a walk. These are what bring me joy. And the rest I am still trying to figure it out'.

Nina

'Having cancer brought some positive things into my life. In particular, I've rid my life of negative people and negative energy and I feel so much lighter as a result'.

Sara

'When I compare my pre-cancer life to the life I'm living now, I can see that today I'm so much more aware, more present, more patient, much happier, calmer and generally full of gratitude. I also experience feelings of real joy which I didn't have before cancer. I've had to work at this. I've used a combination of mindfulness, meditation and yoga to get back in touch with my physical body and the way it's in tune with my mind. I feel more at ease now than I ever have'.

Rachel L

'I'm definitely a different person since having had cancer. I think that it gave me the confidence to start a number of new things in my life – things that I probably wouldn't have done if I hadn't had cancer: I've changed jobs, I've started running, I've joined a rock choir and I've joined two book clubs'.

Rachel B

'Since having cancer my attitude has changed. I put myself first a lot more now and I choose whether I can be bothered with something or not, rather than just going along with it. I've taken steps to make my life a lot less stressful and I'm making the most out of life'.

Julie

'I have rediscovered my love of art and being creative, and I paint most days. Art is my therapy'.

Laura

'You can't go through something like cancer without a shift in the way you think. I now grab any opportunity to live life to the max'.

Vicky

'My perspective on life has changed since cancer. I now feel like I want to live my life rather than just existing. If I want to do something, I now just go and do it'.

Jo H

'I know times of crisis can cause people to question their faith but cancer has made me surer of what I believe'.

Laura

'My spirituality has always been important to me, but since having breast cancer I've come to realise that it really is the backbone of my life'.

Toni-Ann

Top tips

- Simplify your life
- Stop overthinking
- Stay in the present
- Let go of the bad stuff
- Practise kindness and gratitude
- Have patience
- Don't compare yourself to others
- Slow down
- Live your life and don't just exist
- Don't sweat the small stuff
- Don't worry what other people think
- Stay balanced
- Be yourself
- Move forward step by step, one day at a time
- Live, don't exist

Notes

What are your reflections on life, the world and how you fit into it?

The toolkit

'I need to stop. I need to press the pause button. I need to take a few deep breaths and I need to think about how to get through this'.

Taken from Ticking Off Breast Cancer

Welcome to the Toolkit. This section is all about building the tools and strategies for your own recovery toolkit: finding the things that help you to process what you've been through, what you're currently going through and where you're moving onto. Throughout the book, you will have seen a number of suggestions for coping with the various challenges covered in the book. These are:

- Breathing exercises
- Mindfulness exercises
- Journalling and writing
- Keeping a gratitude journal
- Affirmations
- A healthy bedtime routine

Essentially, they're all suggestions for ways in which you can practise self-care, and whilst this Toolkit focuses on these, there are many other ways of practising self-care. Essentially it comes down to treating yourself kindly and with compassion. Try to carve out some time for yourself every day when you can do something that makes you feel good:

Have a cuppa	Have a rest
Go for a walk	Do some colouring
Chat to a friend	Cuddle a pet
Do some exercise	Sing
Spend time in nature	Say no
Listen to music	Go to bed early
Put on a face treatment mask	Have a nap
Potter in the garden	Do a yoga class
Dance	Make a healthy meal
Unplug electronics	Do a guided meditation
Read a book	Get some fresh air
Have a bubble bath	Be creative
Have a glass of water	Bake some goodies
Listen to a podcast	

I should point out that your recovery toolkit is individual to you. It's not a one-size-fits-all situation. You need to work out what works for you and to do this I suggest that – over time – you give each of these tools a go. Maybe don't try everything all at once – that might be a little overwhelming. Instead, maybe you could try incorporating a couple into your life at a time. When trying out a tool, practise it for a little while. You might not notice the benefits immediately. Be patient and take your time.

It's good practice to incorporate a few tools into daily life going forward and not just until you're 'feeling better'. There will always be challenges in life and having a toolkit of self-care tools that you know work for you, will help you in the long run. However, before we look at each of these tools in detail, let's take a moment to talk about self-care generally.

Self-care isn't being selfish and it's not being indulgent. It's also not just about things like having a bubble bath by candlelight once in a while or going to a spa for some treatments (although both of these are very lovely and are part of what self-care is all about). Self-care is more than the odd treat for yourself. Self-care is practising, on a regular basis, caring for yourself. It's about looking out for, and looking after, your mind and body whilst listening to the needs of your mind and body. It's about taking care to maintain a healthy mind and body and if something isn't quite right; it's about identifying what's going on, what you need and then doing something about it. For example, if you're tired, then rest or have a nap; if you're feeling anxious, consider what you can do to address the anxiety rather than pushing it down or ignoring it; and if you're experiencing continual discomfort or pain, see a doctor rather than hoping it will go away.

Self-care is about eating a healthy diet, getting a good night's sleep, getting enough good quality exercise, having time to yourself, getting fresh air, having the time to process your thoughts, drinking enough water, recognizing when you need to take a break, addressing any feelings of anxiety or stress, talking to someone when you need to and not rushing around at a hundred miles an hour.

In the context of life after cancer, self-care is all about taking action to physically, emotionally and mentally recover from your cancer diagnosis and treatment, and then to maintain your physical, emotional and mental health going forward.

Incorporating self-care into daily life will help every aspect of your recovery. Let me give you three examples. Exercise will, among other things, help improve anxiety, menopausal side-effects, fatigue, lymphoedema and reduce the risk of recurrence. Mindfulness will help reduce stress and feelings of anxiety, whilst also helping to cope with the fear of recurrence. And writing or journalling has the potential to help you cope with all the challenges you face as a result of having had cancer whilst helping you move forward in your life.

Many of us go through life putting ourselves at the bottom of the priority list, but we need to move ourselves up the list. We need to look after ourselves so that we can look after and out for everyone else: partners, children, parents and friends. Remember, you can't pour from an empty cup.

Breathing exercises

'Close your eyes and take a few deep breaths'.

Taken from Ticking Off Breast Cancer

Breathing exercises help lower the stress in your body because when you breathe deeply, it sends a message to your brain to calm down and relax and the brain then sends a message to your body to calm down and relax. They can be particularly effective when you are feeling anxious, especially if you're experiencing a physiological response to the anxiety – such as a racing heart, butterflies in your tummy or feeling shaky. Breathing exercises can also be used on a daily basis – for example, for a couple of minutes when you wake up in the morning. Practising them on a daily basis can help to reduce anxiety and stress. You can do breathing exercises anywhere and you only need a few minutes for them to be effective.

A breathing exercise for when you are on the go

1 Stop what you're doing.
2 You can either stand or sit.
3 Put your hand on your stomach.
4 Take a deep breath in.

5 Slowly release your breath.

6 Repeat five times.

7 Focus on your breath throughout.

Breathing exercises for when you have a little more time

1 Sit down if possible.

2 Take five deep breaths in and out.

3 Bring yourself back to the present.

4 Say, I'm present in the here and now. I'm okay right at this minute.

5 Repeat a few times until you feel calmer.

1 Sit down or lie down somewhere quiet.

2 Close your eyes if it feels comfortable to do so.

3 Breathe deeply in and out.

4 Just notice the breath going in and out, in and out, in and out...

5 Notice where there is tension in your body and breathe into those places.

1 Sit down or lie down somewhere quiet.

2 Close your eyes if it feels comfortable to do so.

3 Breathe naturally.

4 Focus on your breath.

5 Count your breaths up to ten and then count your breaths back down from ten.

6 Repeat if necessary.

More information about breathing exercises

If you want to learn more, you can find breathing exercises on Apps for your phone, YouTube and online. Why not make a cup of tea and spend some time exploring these to find something that you feel would work for you?

Mindfulness

'Look around you. Notice the trees, the sky, what's going on and remind yourself that right here and now you're alright'.

Taken from Ticking Off Breast Cancer

Many of the emotions and feelings experienced after cancer treatment can be incredibly daunting. It's easy to feel like your head is awash with a myriad of complex thoughts and emotions whilst your body mirrors those feelings with a raft of physiological symptoms such as headaches, butterflies in your tummy and a racing heart. Add in trying to cope with everything that regular life throws at you after treatment – back to work, back to the school run and back to life – with little energy, plenty of fatigue and regular sleepless nights, and you can feel majorly stressed, upset and overwhelmed.

So, wouldn't it be helpful to find something that you could do to help calm your anxious mind and stressed-out body? Particularly if you could do it anywhere; for free; for five minutes or fifty-five minutes; and on your own, or as part of a group. This is where mindfulness comes in.

Mindfulness is a simple process by which you bring a sense of present moment awareness with your breath and senses, developing your ability to pay attention to what is going on around you internally and externally, in the present moment and non-judgmentally. Doing simple mindfulness exercises and living your day-to-day life in a mindful way, can be helpful in reducing the ability of your thoughts to consume you. Mindfulness doesn't take away the difficult thoughts like the fear of a cancer recurrence or the anxiety about what you've been through, but it instead allows you to live calmly alongside such thoughts.

With the insight and advice of Laura Ashurst, who is an accredited Breathworks mindfulness teacher, this section of the Toolkit will give you some background about mindfulness and how it can help you, together with some simple exercises you can do on your own.

What is mindfulness? How does it help?

- Mindfulness is a way of calming the mind and body by staying in the present moment.
- Mindfulness helps to bring a sense of awareness of the present moment – rather than focusing on what's happened in the past; what might happen in the future; and all the 'what-ifs' running around in your head.
- Mindfulness gives you some breathing space: it can slow down a racing heartbeat, it can calm the tingling in your chest and it can give you a fresh perspective on your worries.

- Mindfulness helps reduce the ruminating, catastrophic thinking and the worrying associated with going over the same thing again and again and again.
- Mindfulness cultivates an ability to step back from your thoughts and to understand that you are not your thoughts: thoughts are often not facts but rather they are the story you create in your mind about a situation.
- Mindfulness encourages you to pause and tune into your mind and body, breaking the cycle of over-thinking and associated physiological symptoms.
- Mindfulness enables you to recognize when your brain has strayed into troublesome thought patterns and encourages you to take a step back from them.
- Mindfulness is not about telling yourself to be positive – it's about helping you to identify how you feel in the present moment and then, as and when needed if you're struggling, is useful as a tool to help you deal with difficult situations.
- Mindfulness is not about blocking out pain, anxiety or stress – it's about acknowledging that you are feeling a particular way but that you don't need to attach yourself to these feelings.

Let me give you an example. Say you've got a scan coming up. It's very easy to focus your thoughts on this upcoming scan and your mind can easily jump on the thought train in the direction of getting bad results and having to go through another cancer diagnosis, treatment and all the stress associated with that. You could be picturing the consultant giving you the news and you might see yourself telling the children. But it doesn't stop there, these thoughts keep going round and round in your head and you start to feel sick and unable to eat, your heart is racing and you have a headache.

By practising mindfulness – doing a simple exercise or one of the daily life mindfulness practices – you will notice that you are allowing your thoughts to get carried away and that it's having a physiological impact on you. You'll be able to recognize that you're worried about the scan but you'll be able to take a step back from these thoughts and bring yourself into the present moment, breaking the cycle of catastrophic thinking.

Mindfulness exercises

There are lots of mindfulness exercises, mindfulness meditations, and mindfulness practices that you can incorporate into your daily life. Here are three simple mindfulness exercises, recommended by Laura, that you can practise at home. You can practise these when you are feeling stressed or anxious, or you can get into the habit of practising them on a regular basis regardless of how you feel at that moment.

1 Pause, just for a few minutes, to notice how you are feeling and to check in with your breathing. Creating moments in the day where you are choosing to actively stop what you are doing to ask yourself how you are feeling, allows the pause button on the busyness of the day to be pressed. This act is a self-care strategy that seems very simplistic but it allows you to notice areas of tension in the body and the pattern of your breath. Simply notice without judgment and then breathe in and out for one minute, without forcing the breath in any way, just noticing the flow of the breath as it moves in and out of your body.

2 Ground yourself by noticing how the floor beneath you is supporting your feet. This can be done anywhere, at any time. In a seated position, as you notice your feet being supported, also notice how the surface that you are sitting on is supporting you. Take a moment to allow your body to sink into gravity a little further, by allowing the surface beneath you to support you fully.

3 Actively choose to notice sounds in your immediate environment. Becoming more fully aware of sounds in the space that you're in, helps to give a sense of connection with your environment. You don't need to label them as something that you like or dislike. You are simply choosing to acknowledge them, tuning your ears into the sounds. Focusing your attention in this way helps to develop awareness of what's around you.

Bringing mindfulness into daily life

Mindfulness isn't just about doing the exercises once in a while, when you're feeling stressed or anxious, or even on a daily basis. It's also about living more mindfully: moving yourself from the busyness of 'doing mode' where you are constantly analysing, problem solving, evaluating and over-thinking, towards a calmer 'being mode' where you perform things on a slower, more thoughtful basis: carrying out one activity at a time with an awareness of the breath and your senses. According to Laura, the benefits of 'being mode' are that it helps to dampen down your stress response; lowers adrenaline and cortisol levels; and increases the output of the neurotransmitters, endorphins and serotonin, helping to make you feel calmer and more settled. In turn, lowering the levels of adrenaline and cortisol, it helps you to cope with difficult situations and thought processes as and when they arise.

Laura's advice is that by incorporating mindfulness into daily life, you'll benefit in subtle ways that become more apparent with regular practice: an ability to think more clearly by becoming less caught up in negative thought processes. You will feel more energized which can lead to enhanced levels of creativity and an ability to become more aware of what's happening moment-to-moment, in both your internal and external environment. Mindfulness isn't going to solve all of your problems but it will help you to respond to them in a way that's less reactive.

Here are Laura's suggestions for some simple ways to bring mindfulness into your daily life:

A mindful walk

Walking is such a great exercise option on many levels, especially post-cancer. You're increasing the oxygen being taken into your body and you're taking in essential vitamin D. Walking also strengthens bones (useful for those of you going through the menopause or who are on hormone therapy and at risk of osteoarthritis); it can help control lymphoedema swelling; it helps to expend calories (again this is helpful for those of you experiencing weight gain as a result of chemotherapy or hormone therapy); eases joint pain (another side-effect of hormone therapy), helps with fatigue and can boost your mood. And, if you choose to walk mindfully, then you'll also benefit from the positive effects of mindfulness.

Walking mindfully involves using all your senses to become more aware of the experience of the walk, rather than allowing your thoughts to run away so that you are spending the walk thinking about worst case scenarios and scary 'what-if' situations. As you're walking, consider the following:

1 What can you feel? How does your posture change as you propel yourself forwards? How does your foot feel as you step down onto your heel and lift off from the ball of your foot? How does the ground feel? What is the temperature and how does the air feel on your exposed skin?

2 Look around you. What can you see with your mindful gaze that you may not have noticed before? How does the sunlight make the buildings look? How do the shadows look on the ground before you? If you're in a rural location, notice the trees, the sky, and the horizon. If you're in a built-up location, notice the brickwork and structure of the buildings, the sky and the reflections in the windows.

3 What can you hear? Actively listen to the sounds around you. Can you hear birdsong? How many different types of bird? What about traffic? People talking? The crunching of the dirt underfoot as you take each step?

4 What smells do you notice? Can you smell freshly cut grass? A bonfire? Blossom on the tree? Wet grass after rainfall?

5 It can help to 'walk with five': think about five things you can feel, see, hear, smell and touch.

Mindful eating

Mindful eating is all about focusing on your meal and the process of eating, rather than thinking about the list of things you still have to do over the remainder of the day, the scan that's coming up, or focusing on the anxious post-cancer thoughts running through your mind. And there's an added health benefit – eating mindfully allows the gut to recognize when it's full, thus allowing you to avoid over-eating.

Simply focus on the food as you eat it, using all of your senses. Notice how the food looks as it sits in the bowl or on the plate. What shapes, colours and smells are present? Notice how cutlery feels in your hand and as you bring the food towards your mouth, pause again to notice its smell and texture. Look at the food, noticing once more its shape and colour before the food is placed in your mouth. As you move it around your mouth with your tongue and your teeth, notice the texture and taste of the food and the sound of it being moved around your mouth as you chew and swallow the food.

Slowing down the whole process of taking food into our bodies in this way helps us to awaken the senses and focus on the act of eating; it helps us to become more aware of each mouthful of food and for the brain to acknowledge when our stomach feels full.

Mindful bathing

We wash our body so regularly that we can carry out this activity on autopilot without having to think about what we are doing. Being on autopilot is an opportunity for us to be mindless and for our minds to become so lost in thought that we miss the whole process of whatever activity it is that we are doing! On the other hand, mindful bathing or showering creates an opportunity to focus our senses on the single act of washing our bodies. It helps us to move away from the busyness of our thoughts and to create moments where our senses allow our mind to focus on one single activity.

Focusing our attention and awareness on our senses during a bath or shower turns the process into a mindful activity where you can actively notice when your thoughts have drifted to other things. With an air of gentle kindness, you can encourage yourselves with your breathing and the use of your senses to return to the activity of washing: the sound, touch and temperature of the water on your skin, the smell of the soap or shower gel and its texture and sound as you use it to clean your body. Noticing how you are being supported by the surface beneath you helps to create further awareness of your body. The sensation of the fabric of the flannel or shower mitt on your skin, along with the towel that you use at the end of your bathing experience is another texture-based experience for your senses to absorb and notice.

Habits

We are all creatures of habit but many of the things that we do habitually don't serve us well. For example, habitually being caught up in past and future thinking increases our levels of anxiety: this leads us to continually over-react to things without giving ourselves time to respond in a more measured way, thus creating situations where we berate ourselves afterwards. Over-indulging with food and alcohol can easily lead to habitual patterns where we are unkind to ourselves afterwards as a result of our behaviour. Mindfulness helps us to make healthier life choices by encouraging moments where we pause to take a breath, taking a physical and mental step back and becoming more mindfully aware of our actions.

Recognizing how you are feeling, encourages you to notice that it's your stress levels that are often leading you to make particular choices. Taking the time to reflect on your choices and how a particular course of action makes you feel afterwards creates some space between you and the next step. Will your habitual choice nourish and nurture you helping you to thrive or will it serve to make you feel more anxious and unhappy with yourself afterwards? Habits can be so ingrained within us that, often, we've taken a course of action without even thinking about it.

Life after active treatment for primary breast cancer presents many challenges but it also presents opportunities for you to make mindful choices about your patterns of behaviour. What are the triggers to your habits? Can they be explored and supported in a more nurturing way?

Is it possible for you to take several breaths in and several breaths out to create a moment of mindfulness and a pause where you can consider your next step? Actively choosing to take another route with your choices helps to reduce habitual patterns of behaviour. Mindfulness helps to create moments of self-care; moments where the actions that you take are ones that serve to bolster and boost your well-being. It also helps you to be more kind to yourselves in your decision-making processes.

More information about mindfulness

If you want to learn more about mindfulness, there's a lot of information available on the internet and by way of books (see the Useful Resources section for some recommendations). If you'd like to develop your mindfulness, you can take mindfulness classes, join mindfulness groups, take a course in mindfulness and follow mindfulness meditations on the internet.

To end this section on mindfulness, I'd like to share Laura's poem – 'You Who Lives; A Self-Judging Being' – which sums up what mindfulness is all about.

You, who lives; a self-judging being,

You, who has lived through so much unseen.

You, who listens to your thoughts and lets them dwell

In your heart, yet they don't feed or serve you well.

Our breath is there to soothe like a balm,

In quiet and loud times, helping calm.

Step back from the judgement of your inner thought

Watch it pass on by noticing how it sought

To make you believe you aren't enough,

Making you feel small when life gets tough.

Open your wings and let them gently unfurl,

That thought isn't you, with its stealthy swirl.

Pause, just notice its presence, and then

With your next breath out, simply watch it when,

It passes on by, with permission from you

Making room for self–growth, for you to renew,

Yourself, each breath, each moment, again,

Start over, climb off the judgement train.

You, in every part of your beautiful soul

Has the strength to face all emotional toll.

Breathe in, breath out; don't make it a fight.

Let judgement subside, feeling the light,

You, here and now, the breath breathing all of you

Over and over, each moment begins new.

Journalling and writing prompts

'Writing enables me to take all the chaotic, confused, anxious thoughts that are crowding my brain and put them into some sort of structured order'.

Taken from Ticking Off Breast Cancer

Using writing to help you process what you've been through, what you're currently going through and where you wish to go, can take various forms: journalling, writing, creative writing, mind dumps, keeping a gratitude journal and using a worry jar. This part of the Toolkit guides you through all of these with the aim of getting you started on a writing journey. There are plenty of books and resources dedicated to writing and journalling, some of which are recommended in the Useful Resources section of this book. It's also worth noting that writing doesn't work for everyone, but it's one of those things that's worth trying. Take me as an example, I was never a writer or diary-keeper, but when I turned to writing as a way to cope with having been through cancer, I never turned back.

Journalling

Journalling is the practice of writing about your experiences, emotions and feelings on a regular basis – ideally every day. You can write about anything and everything that comes into your head – so this will include how you're currently feeling and what you're currently doing, as well as exploring what you went through with cancer and how that made you feel. So, in the aftermath of cancer, journalling can help you process all those feelings and emotions that you're experiencing: anxiety, trauma, sadness, grief, loss of confidence, distress and everything else. Journalling is a great way of organizing and processing that tangled jumble of thoughts, emotions and feelings that you're experiencing right now.

It's good to get in the practice of journalling every day and many people find it helpful to do it either just before going to bed or as soon as they get up in the morning. Allie Morgan – the Confidence Coach who has talked us through many of the challenges in this book – says:

'One of the first things I do when I wake up is write in my journal. It's the best time of the day for me to focus and think about what I want the day ahead to hold for me. As an early bird, I'm currently waking up while the mornings are still dark and I find journalling with a cup of tea really helps to set me up for the day ahead'.

A worry jar

A worry jar is a jar into which you put your worries. Find yourself a jar with a lid and some small pieces of paper. Then, whenever you're worried, anxious, stressed, angry or upset about something, you write it down on a piece of paper and pop it into the jar. This is a simple way of taking these thoughts out of your head and putting them somewhere else.

Creative writing

Creative writing involves writing stories, essays and poetry whilst exploring your feelings in an indirect way. You could write a short story about someone who's been through cancer, a poem about an aspect of cancer or a piece of prose about a defining memory that you have. The writing doesn't necessarily have to be about you or your experience but in using this form of writing as therapy, invariably you'll be using your experiences, emotions and feelings as the basis of your writing. There are online classes, in-person classes, books and websites all dedicated to using creative writing as therapy – some are listed in the Useful Resources section of the book.

Writing

Some people want to specifically write about what they've been through during cancer, rather than journalling every day or writing creatively. This type of writing practice can be a helpful way to process the emotions and feelings that you've experienced and are continuing to experience. Again, it's a way to process everything that's crowding your brain. You don't need to write every day; you just write when you feel up to it.

This practice of writing involves writing about what you've been through, what you're going through and your future goals. If you feel up to it, it's good practice to think about all three areas in your writing, because this will help get all the emotions, thoughts and feelings out of you and onto the paper where they have less power over you.

Writing about what you've been through allows you to take an experience over which you have had no, or little, control – which was thus completely overwhelming and very scary – and to put it into some sort of structured order on paper or your computer screen. This enables you to regain some sort of control over the cancer situation, making it less overwhelming and less scary. It's like Dr Jane Clark says in Chapter 7, processing trauma by regularly talking about what you've been through allows the memory of your experience to lose its intensity, and similarly, writing about a traumatic experience can also help minimize the emotional intensity of that experience allowing you to process it.

Writing about how you're currently feeling and what is currently going on in your life can also be very therapeutic as it allows you to take stock of where you are. It gives you some breathing space: your head might be full of all sorts of emotions – like the ones covered in this book – and in order to process what you're currently going through, you need to process those emotions and feelings. Writing them out onto a piece of paper or onto your computer screen can help you to look at them in a different light, put them into some sort of order and understand what you need to do to help yourself deal with them.

Writing about your future goals and plans is a great way to look forward to a brighter future. Don't be scared to have hopes, dreams and plans. This is the exciting part.

Mind dump

You could start writing – whether you're going to be journalling, creative writing or writing about what you've been through – with a 'mind dump'. This is where you sit with a blank sheet of paper (or ideally a few sheets – perhaps a notebook) and write down everything that comes into your head. To get started, write out words on a piece of paper like, chemo, hair loss, diagnosis, children, partner, friends... Words that relate to you and your situation. Then look at all the words and think about how you relate to that word and how each word makes you feel. You can just think in your head, or you can write notes at this stage. What usually happens is that one or two of those words will stand out to you more than the others – you'll be drawn to thinking/writing about them more than the others. You can then write about those topics. Throw down sentences, words and phrases in no order. This 'mind dump' can help get lots of muddled anxious thoughts out of your head. You can then move on to write about some of these things in a more structured way, which might help you regain control over them.

Getting started

There are no rules for journalling or writing about your experience. Nothing is off limits. To get you started here are some tips:

- Taking just five minutes every morning and evening to journal can be a really cathartic experience.
- Remember that you are writing for whatever reason that you choose. So, if you don't want anyone to read what you've written, then they don't have to. Nobody needs to ever read it; you could even ceremoniously destroy it, in a defiant move against cancer.
- Everyone can write about their experience. You don't need to be a writer. You just need a pen and paper, or a laptop, or a phone. You don't need to be perfect at grammar and spelling. Just remember to write what is important to you, write from the heart and be honest with yourself.
- Don't be afraid to write down your feelings and emotions, your fears and worries. If you write them out, then they're out of your head and you can let them go. It might even help lift the weight of anxiety off your chest a little.
- If there's anything you're worrying about, note that down too and see if there's anything you can do about it. Are you able to speak to a doctor or a professional? Can you ask a friend to help?
- Don't forget to write about the good as well as the bad. For example, you could write down some of the good things that happened throughout your day – it can be something simple like going for a walk.
- Try noting down the things you're grateful for, what you'd love to receive, what you want to focus on and how you want to feel at the end of the day. Check out the next section of the Toolkit which gives guidance on writing a gratitude journal.
- You might want to write in a group with others who are in your position or with the guidance of a trained counsellor. Equally, you can choose to do it by yourself.
- Here are some writing prompts. You could use a different one each day, or you might find that just using a few to get you started will lead to the writing flowing. You don't need to start at the top of the list and work your way through, have a look at the list and choose the prompts that appeal to you the most.

Writing about your diagnosis and treatment

Write about how you were diagnosed with cancer – what's your diagnosis story?

How did you feel to be diagnosed with cancer?

What were the key moments of your diagnosis?

How did it feel to tell your parents, siblings, children that you had cancer?

What was the hardest part of your diagnosis; how did you deal with it?

How did your friends treat you when you told them about your diagnosis?

Write about having treatment for cancer – what is your treatment story?

How did you feel about losing your hair through chemotherapy?

What was the hardest part of your treatment; how did you deal with it?

How did your friends treat you as you were going through treatment?

What side-effects did you experience and how did you cope with them?

Complete the sentence:

I remember...

I was scared when...

It made me sad when...

Writing about the changes you've experienced as a result of having had cancer

Write a letter to the person you were before cancer. What words of advice would you give and what would you say to that person? Perhaps you would say things like:

I'm grateful to you for ...

I'll miss ... about you.

I think about you and I remember ...

Thank you for ...

I'm sorry for ...

I've changed now ...

If you could go back in time ten years, what advice would you give yourself?

How has having cancer changed you as a person?

What physical changes have you experienced? How do they make you feel?

What have you learnt about yourself since being diagnosed with cancer?

How have your relationships (with family and friends) changed since you've been diagnosed with cancer?

Have you noticed a change in yourself since the date you were diagnosed? How did you deal with the diagnosis? With the treatment? And now that treatment has ended?

What has been your biggest challenge since finishing your treatment? How did you cope with it?

How do you see your 'new normal'? How do you feel about starting a 'new normal'?

What is important to you?

Complete the sentences:

Before I was diagnosed with cancer, I wish I'd known ...

The things I learnt from having cancer are ...

Writing about the here and now: how you're feeling and what you're going through

If someone you really care about was in your position right now, what words of comfort and encouragement would you give them?

What are you grateful for today?

How are you feeling today? Right now, at this very moment?

When was the last time you felt angry?

When was the last time you felt sad?

When was the last time you felt content?

What happened today and how do you feel about it?

What has cancer made you realize, that perhaps you didn't before?

What would you like to say to your friends and family but you feel you can't? Can you write a letter to them explaining how you feel? You don't need to send the letter.

Here are some words to prompt your writing. How do you feel when you read these words? Have you felt these emotions recently? Can you write about when you felt these emotions?

Hopeful	Content	Weak
Lonely	Happy	Identity
Loved	Grateful	Loss
Scared	Stressed	
Worried	Strong	

Complete the sentence (and continue writing on this theme):

Today I feel …
I am most grateful for …
Today I choose to feel …
I find joy in …
I am good at …
I can …
I feel like I have lost …
I am grieving for …
I'm finding it hard to …

Writing about your goals and plans

What has changed since cancer?
How are you different since cancer?
What are your priorities now?
How has your perspective changed on the things in your life?
What do you want from your life?
What are you appreciative of?
What are you grateful for?
What have you learnt by going through cancer?
What is important to you?
If you could change one thing about your life after cancer, what would it be and why?
What is your no. 1 goal for the next year?
Complete the sentence …

My plans for the future are …
I would like to …

> I dream of ...
> I hope to ...

Just a little note about writing and journalling. Do be aware that writing about what you've been through can be quite triggering so it's important to do it in a safe, comfortable environment. If you think it might be hard to write about some aspects of your cancer experience it might be worth approaching those with friends, others in a support group or a counsellor.

A gratitude journal

'Life is not a competition or about striving for perfection or worrying about what other people think. It's about appreciating what I have, not thinking about what I want next'.

Taken from Ticking Off Breast Cancer

The human brain is wired to focus on the negative. This is because the negatives are most likely to threaten survival and the brain's number one job is to ensure survival – everything else comes second. Dr Jane Clark told me:

'It's helpful to think of negative thoughts like motorways in the brain; they are well developed pathways so they are quicker to recall. So, we need to focus our attention on – and rehearse – the positives in order to balance this out. The positives are often like little country lanes: by repeating them, we strengthen these pathways in the brain into proper roads'.

It's therefore important to find ways to break the negative cycle and one way of doing this is to start a gratitude journal.

There are various ways of writing a gratitude journal and you can even buy specific gratitude journals which include writing prompts and suggestions. But all you really need is a notebook and pen and to write a list of the things for which you are grateful at the end/start of each day. It's helpful to aim to write your gratitude journal every day. It can be a nice part of your bedtime routine to focus on the positive things from the day. Or you can start your day by writing your gratitude journal – it's a great way to start the day off on a positive note.

You could start with a basic list of things for which you are grateful. Try listing between three and five things every day. Some days you might find that there are many things to list and other days there won't be quite so many. Think about things you've experienced, such as a lovely walk in the sun, a delicious meal or an enjoyable yoga class. You could include something you've received, such as a phone call from a friend, an invitation or an act of kindness. Try thinking about something you have and which you usually take for granted, such as the love and support of your family and friends. Include people in the list, such as a friend, family member or a kind stranger. You might find it difficult to start with, so here are some prompts to get you going:

What was the best part of your day today?
Who have you been grateful for today?
Who was kind to you today?
What did you smile about today?
Who has made you smile recently?
Which friend are you particularly grateful for today?
Have you listened to any uplifting music today?
What three qualities about yourself are you grateful for?
Who are you grateful to have in your life?
What self-care did you practise today?
What went well today?
What did you do today that you are proud of?
What are you looking forward to?
When did you feel gratitude today?
What insight did you gain today?
What beauty did you see today?
Did you overcome any challenges today?
How did you show yourself kindness today?
What did you learn today?
What is going well for you at the moment?
What or who has made you happy today?
Which positive emotions did you experience today?
Describe one of your strengths for which you are grateful.

Affirmations

'You can achieve things if you put your mind to it'.

Taken from Ticking Off Breast Cancer

As you've just read in the section on writing a gratitude journal, our brains are wired to think negatively so we need to focus on positive thoughts. Affirmations are short, simple, positive statements designed to help you reduce a negative thought pattern that you may find yourself in as a result of experiencing some complex and distressing emotions and feelings after cancer. The words in the statement bring up positive images and these help to motivate you into changing the way you think and act.

It's helpful to choose two or three affirmations relevant to your current personal situation and repeat them first thing in the morning as you start your day, and last thing at night when you go to bed. You can write them on little sticky notes and attach them to you mirror, fridge door or inside a cupboard that you regularly open. Repeat them a few times with confidence and belief in yourself. And do this, with the same affirmations, for a couple of weeks or even longer. You can make up your own affirmations to suit your personal goals, but here are some suggestions:

I am enough just as I am
I am not defined by cancer
I am worthy
I am valuable
I am loved
I am strong
I'm grateful for my body's resilience
I will take each day as it comes
I will allow myself time to rest
Being kind to myself is my priority
I have a beautiful life ahead of me
I am in charge of my future
I will make my life everything I want it to be
I am grateful for my supportive family/friends
I deserve to be happy
I deserve to be loved
I forgive my body

My body is strong and healthy
I deserve love and respect
I am choosing happiness today

A healthy bedtime routine

'I can get very busy in the pitch black of night, asking question after question, rarely coming up with any answers and constantly searching for peace of mind'.

Taken from Ticking Off Breast Cancer

Yes, I know that you are fully aware of what makes a healthy bedtime routine – you can read about this on a daily basis in all the lifestyle magazines and across social media. But I'm going to repeat it all here because a key to coping with the challenges you face after cancer treatment is getting a good night's sleep. This can often feel impossible given the hot flushes, discomfort from surgery and the 3 a.m. thought train into the land of worry and anxiety. But if you can incorporate a healthy routine then it will go a long way to getting some of the very important sleep that both your body and mind need.

What is hindering your sleep?

Look at what's stopping you from falling asleep in the first place or keeping you awake in the middle of the night. If it's pain or discomfort then you need to address this by talking to your doctor or your medical team. For example, physiotherapy might help post-surgery pain; scar tissue massage might soothe surgical scars; and manual lymphatic drainage might help with uncomfortable lymphoedema.

If you're experiencing night sweats or hot flushes as a result of hormone treatment or a medically induced menopause, consider making yourself more comfortable by having a small can of water spray and a fan by your bed, using a cooling pillow and wearing nightwear that's designed for women experiencing night sweats. For example, you can get bamboo nightwear which is highly breathable, absorbent and temperature regulating.

Now address your sleeping area. Is the room dark enough? Do you need to get some blackout lining for your curtains or would an eye mask help? How is your mattress and pillow? Are you sleeping next to a snorer and would earplugs help? Are you warm enough or cool enough at night?

Can you adjust the radiator controls? Do you need to change from one heavy bed covering to layered covers that you can remove or add over the course of the night? Do you charge your phone by your bed and if so, can you move the charger outside your room?

Do you wake up in the night?

Do you wake up in the night with your mind racing about things you've forgotten to do and things you need to remember to do? In order to avoid this happening, it can be helpful to spend a few moments at the end of the day, before getting ready for bed, going through what you've done today and what your plans are for tomorrow.

You can make a list of the things you need to remember to do the following day and then you can prepare for bed in the knowledge that everything is under control. It might help to have a notepad and pen next to your bed just in case you still wake in the night remembering, for example, that you haven't collected the dry cleaning. But by getting into the habit of doing this review of the day/plan for tomorrow, the less you'll need your notebook in the middle of the night.

Do you wake up in the night with your mind racing with anxious thoughts? Have you hopped on the thought train to the land of anxiety where you're jumping ahead of yourself and thinking about all sorts of horrible what-if scenarios? The mind can be so powerful that, lying there in the middle of the night, you'll start believing that this little journey is the truth. The key here is to recognize right at the start of this little thought train, that your mind is going off on a little fictional journey and that you need to bring it back to the here and now. As you lie there, try one of the breathing exercises or mindfulness exercises set out in the previous sections of the Toolkit.

Your bedtime routine

And now, after addressing all the other factors that are affecting your ability to get a good night's sleep, it's time to think about your bedtime routine.

- Try to avoid screens for a while before you go to bed – yes, you know this already but maybe you need a little reminder!
- Create a calming bedtime environment with, for example, calming music, soft lighting and using a bedtime pillow spray (these are available from many places and contain calming essential oils such as lavender).

- Sometimes a warm relaxing bath can help switch off from the day and prepare your mind and body for sleep. Consider using some bath salts or bath oil which help promote relaxation like ones with lavender oil.
- Think about what you are grateful for and what went well during your day. Going to sleep with a positive mindset can help avoid those negative thoughts that keep you awake.
- Try listening to a guided meditation – it will help you to switch off from the day and prepare you for sleep.
- As you lie in bed trying to sleep, try one of the simple breathing exercises described in the Breathing Exercises section of the Toolkit, or do a body scan:
  - Take a few deep breathes in through your nose and slowly out through your mouth.
  - Now, in your mind, start a scan of your body to identify areas of tension which you can then switch off and relax.
  - Start with your feet. How do your toes and the soles of your feet feel? How do your ankles feel? Relax the muscles in your feet and move up to your calves and shins – how do they feel? Relax the muscles and move up to your knees.
  - You get the picture – keep doing this all the way up your body paying special attention to areas of tension such as your stomach, back, shoulders, neck, top of your head and jawline (relax your mouth by moving your tongue to the bottom of your mouth).

Useful resources

Top of my list of useful resources is the online support hub of the **Future Dreams Breast Cancer Charity** website: www.futuredreams.org.uk. I run this site together with a team of women who – just like you – have had primary breast cancer. In addition to providing information and support to people going through treatment, a lot of what we do is aimed at people – like you – who have finished their treatment and are now navigating their way through post-cancer life.

And now, in alphabetical order, are some places where you will find information, advice and support on the issues covered in this book.

Anxiety and trauma

- The **Blurt Foundation** is a social enterprise dedicated to helping those affected by depression. The have a brilliant website with loads of resources: www.blurtitout.org.
- **Breast Cancer Now** have a section on their website about managing stress and anxiety: www.breastcancernow.org/information-support/facing-breast-cancer/living-beyond-breast-cancer/life-after-breast-cancer-treatment/coping-emotionally/managing-stress-anxiety.
- The **BRiC Centre** research aims to reduce the traumatic impact of diagnosis and harsh treatments including the classic chemo brain which is associated with anxiety and depression, to better the quality of life of women with breast cancer: www.briccentre.co.uk.
- **Cancer Research UK** have a page about anxiety: www.cancerresearchuk.org/about-cancer/coping/emotionally/cancer-and-your-emotions/fear-anxiety-panic/about.
- **Macmillan** have a stack of information and advice about dealing with anxiety and cancer: www.macmillan.org.uk/cancer-information-and-support/impacts-of-cancer/anxiety.
- **Trekstock** have an anxiety Q&A with Emily Hodge, MSc Health Psychology, Accredited Coach and Therapist: www.trekstock.com/anxiety.
- **Trekstock** have a selection of videos on their website about coping with anxiety and cancer: www.youtube.com/c/Trekstock.

BAME support organizations

- **Black Women Rising** is a cancer support group based in London, whose mission is to educate, inspire and bring opportunities for women from the BAME community, to connect with one another and share their stories, without fear or shame. They host in person and online support groups, have an annual magazine and a podcast: www.blackwomenrisinguk.org.

Charities

These national charities all provide dedicated support to people who have finished treatment for primary cancer.

- **Breast Cancer Now** have a helpline and a dedicated section on their website on life after breast cancer: www.breastcancernow.org/information-support/facing-breast-cancer/living-beyond-breast-cancer/life-after-breast-cancer-treatment.
- **Macmillan** have a dedicated section on their website for life after cancer: www.macmillan.org.uk/cancer-information-and-support/after-treatment.
- **Maggies** is a charity providing free cancer support and information in centres across the UK and online: www.maggies.org.
- **Penny Brohn** is a national charity providing online zoom sessions on things like mindfulness and breathwork, one-to-one counselling, self-care resources and a range of informative webinars: www.pennybrohn.org.uk.
- **Shine** is a charity which supports adults in their 20s, 30s and 40s with, and beyond, cancer. They have information and advice on their website and they also put on workshops and retreats. They have regional networks which meet in person. They also have private Facebook groups supporting women going through the menopause after cancer and people dating after cancer: www.shinecancersupport.org.
- **Trekstock** supports young adults during/after cancer. They have a wide range of post-cancer support including, a fitness programme, online exercise classes, workshops, in-person meet-ups and more: www.trekstock.com.

- **Wigwam and Yes to Life** is a community of people living with/ beyond cancer coming together to explore and share information and experiences with the aim of empowering themselves to gain control over their lives, focusing on integrated medicine. Wigwam is a place for people to meet locally or online: www.yestolife.org.uk.

Checking your breasts for recurrence/new cancer

- **Coppafeel** is a charity dedicated to helping people check their breasts. They have a host of information on their site and you can sign up for regular reminders to check your breasts. Their website is: www. coppafeel.org.

Chemo brain

- **Cancer Research UK** has helpful advice on their website: www. cancerresearchuk.org/about-cancer/cancer-in-general/treatment/ chemotherapy/side-effects/chemo-brain.
- **Macmillan** have lots of free advice on their website about coping with chemo brain: www.macmillan.org.uk/cancer-information-and- support/impacts-of-cancer/chemo-brain.

Counselling

- **Maggie's** is a charity with support centres situated around the UK. They provide free counselling services.

Exercise

- **5Kyourway** is a community-based initiative to encourage those living with and beyond cancer, families, friends and those working in cancer services to walk, jog, run, cheer or volunteer at a local 5k Your Way parkrun event on the last Saturday of every month. Check out the website to find your nearest parkrun and don't worry about running – you can also walk it: www.5kyourway.org.
- **Breast Cancer Haven** have online videos for all sorts of exercise options including, gentle yoga and Nordic walking: www.breastcan- cerhaven.org.uk.

- **CancerFit** is a website providing resources regarding exercise for people living with and beyond cancer: www.cancerfit.me.
- **Cancer Research UK** provide exercise guidelines for during cancer treatment which are also helpful for someone who has completed treatment: https://www.cancerresearchuk.org/about-cancer/coping/physically/exercise-guidelines.
- **Fighting Fit for Cancer** is an organization offering exercise regimes for people after cancer. It is a fee-paying service but their website is worth checking out for their informative blog: www.ffit4c.com
- **Move Against Cancer** provide lots of support and help in exercising during/after cancer treatment including, for example, a free eight-week online programme: www.movecharity.org.
- **SafeFit** is a research trial designed to support anyone in the UK with suspicion of, or a confirmed diagnosis of, cancer where cancer exercise specialists will offer you free, remote advice, support and resources to maintain and improve physical and emotional well-being: www.safefit.nhs.uk.
- **Trekstock** have loads of information about exercising during and after cancer. The charity specifically supports people in their 20s, 30s and 40s but do still have a look at their resources online if you are older. For those in the right age bracket, RENEW is an amazing free resource – it's their free eight-week group exercise programme, held in London and led by Level 4 Cancer Rehab qualified trainers, and tailored to you. They also offer a great selection of online exercise videos. Check out their website: www.trekstock.com/exercise-cancer.

Fatigue

- **Breast Cancer Now** have lots of free advice on their website about coping with fatigue after breast cancer treatment: www.breastcancernow.org/information-support/facing-breast-cancer/going-through-breast-cancer-treatment/side-effects/fatigue.
- **Macmillan** have lots of free advice on their website about coping with fatigue and tiredness as a result of cancer treatment: www.macmillan.org.uk/cancer-information-and-support/impacts-of-cancer/tiredness.

Fertility

- **Breast Cancer Now** have a section on their website dedicate to fertility issues: www.breastcancernow.org/information-support/facing-breast-cancer/breast-cancer-in-younger-women/fertility-breast-cancer-treatment.

Going back to work

- **Macmillan** have a lot of helpful information on their website dealing with the return to work, your legal rights and so on: www.macmillan.org.uk/cancer-information-and-support/after-treatment/making-decisions-about-work-after-treatment.
- **Working With Cancer** is an organization dedicated to helping people work during cancer treatment or post-cancer treatment. Their services are not free, but their website has a lot of free, helpful information: www.workingwithcancer.co.uk.

Insomnia

- **The Insomniac Clinic** has some useful advice on their website: www.theinsomniaclinic.co.uk.
- **Macmillan** have helpful advice on their website: www.macmillan.org.uk/information-and-support/coping/side-effects-and-symptoms/other-side-effects/difficulty-sleeping.html.

LGBTQIA+ support

- **Live Through This** is a support and advocacy charity for the LGBTIQ+ community. They provide a safe space for anybody who identifies as part of the queer spectrum and has had an experience with any kind of cancer at any stage from testing, diagnosis, treatment, remission to long term care: www.livethroughthis.co.uk.

Lymphoedema

- **British Lymphology Society** is a professional body providing a voice and support for those involved in the care and treatment of people with lymphoedema. Their website contains lots of useful information about lymphoedema including a directory of services around the UK: www.thebls.com.

- **Lymphoedema Support Network** is a charity run by people who live with lymphoedema. Their website provides information for patients about the condition and the experience of living with lymphoedema: www.lymphoedema.org.

Menopause

When reading non-cancer related advice about the menopause, it is important to note that some of the hormone related therapies for dealing with the menopause may not be appropriate for someone who has had breast cancer so it is vitally important to discuss such options with your doctor or oncologist.

- *The Complete Guide to the Menopause: Your Toolkit to Take Control and Achieve Life-Long Health*, **by Dr Annice Mukherjee.** Annice is a hospital medical specialist with a career spanning nearly 30 years. She specializes in general internal medicine and endocrinology with a career-long interest in quality of life in all hormone conditions. She has supported thousands of women going through the menopause, helping them to manage symptoms and improve their quality of life and overall health safely. Her personal experience of an early menopause due to a breast cancer diagnosis gives her a unique perspective and adds to her insight and skills in this field.
- *The Complete Guide to POI and Early Menopause* **by Dr Hannah Short and Dr Mandy Leonhardt** (Sheldon Press, 2022) has some excellent advice on coping with early menopause symptoms – and also on appropriate supplements and support for women who can't take HRT.
- **The Royal Osteoporosis Society** has a lot of helpful advice about bone health even if you haven't developed osteoporosis or osteopenia: www.theros.org.uk.
- **The Menopause and Cancer Podcast from Dani Billington** covers a range of topics related to going through the menopause as a result of cancer treatment including sex after cancer and fertility. It is available from all podcast providers.

Mindfulness

You can go on YouTube and search 'mindfulness'. This brings up loads of guided mindfulness recordings that you can choose from to listen to at home. Specific organizations worth mentioning are:

- **Breathworks** is an organization which provides courses in mindfulness. They also have a directory of mindfulness teachers enabling you to find someone near you: www.breathworks-mindfulness.org.uk.
- **Maggie's** have a good selection of free relaxation videos to choose from: www.maggies.org/cancer-support/managing-emotions/relaxation-and-breathing-exercises.
- **Mindful** is a website which provides lots of advice about mindfulness and meditation: www.mindful.org.
- The **NHS** has a page on mindfulness resources: www.nhs.uk/conditions/stress-anxiety-depression/mindfulness
- Try places like **Balance**, **Headspace** and **Calm** to which you can subscribe and then access daily mindfulness sessions by way of Apps on your phone.
- **Trekstock** give a year's free subscription to Headspace for people in their 20s and 30s with cancer, and **Penny Brohn** give free subscriptions to Headspace.

Moving forward courses

Some charities put on free post-cancer 'moving forward' courses for people who have finished treatment for primary cancer. Some are online and some are in person. Ones to mention are:

- **Breast Cancer Now** have a 'Moving Forward' course for women who have finished breast cancer treatment: www.breastcancernow.org.
- **Life After Cancer** provides a mix of free/paid-for services. They offer support through support groups (online and in person), coaching programmes and one-to-one coaching: www.life-aftercancer.co.uk.
- **Maggie's** put on a 'Where Now?' course: www.maggies.org/cancer-support/our-support/courses-and-workshops/
- **Macmillan** put on a 'HOPE' course at various cancer support centres around the country: https://learnzone.org.uk/courses/course.php?id=111

Nutrition

It's important to get information about nutrition from a registered dietician or nutritionist, particularly one with training in treating people who have had cancer, so check the credentials of anyone from whom you take advice. My recommendations are:

- **Nourish By Jane Clarke** is a website and community dedicated to providing information about nutrition and healthy eating especially for those impacted by illness: www.nourishbyjaneclarke.com.
- **Penny Brohn** have lots of nutrition information on their website: www.pennybrohn.org.uk/.

Parenting

- **Fruitfly Collective** have plenty of resources for parents with cancer. Some of their resources are free and some you need to pay for: www.fruitflycollective.com.
- **Little C Club** is a set of flashcards for children aged 2 years to 10 years to help them understand their parent's cancer diagnosis and treatment: www.littlecclub.com.
- **Macmillan** have plenty of advice for talking to children and teenagers about your cancer. They have a great guide called 'Talking to children and teenagers when an adult has cancer'. https://www.macmillan.org.uk/cancer-information-and-support/diagnosis/talking-about-cancer/talking-to-children-and-teenagers
- The **UK Trauma Council** provides materials on childhood trauma and this would be applicable to children whose parents have cancer. It's geared at people who support children and although you're not doing that, some of the information may be interesting background reading: www.uktraumacouncil.org
- **Cruse Bereavement Care** has some really helpful information about coping with grief: www.cruse.org.uk/get-help/for-parents/childrens-understanding-of-death.
- Barbara Babcock has recommended a book on this topic: *The Book You Wish Your Parents Had Read (and Your Children Will be Glad That You Did)* by Philippa Perry.

Recurrence

- For information about why cancers come back, Cancer Research UK has an informative page: www.cancerresearchuk.org/about-cancer/what-is-cancer/why-some-cancers-come-back.
- For specific advice about breast cancer recurrence, **Breast Cancer Now** have plenty of information on their website, just type 'recurrence' into their search bar: https://breastcancernow.org/

Relationships

All the main charities have advice on their websites about relationship issues arising as a result of cancer. Places like **Maggie's** and **Macmillan** cancer centres also provide free counselling, often for partners as well as patients.

Sleep

- www.helpguide.org have a great selection of articles on getting better sleep.
- www.sleepfoundation.org also have lots of brilliant tips for sleeping better.

Work

- The **Macmillan** website www.macmillan.org.uk has an excellent selection of articles about working after cancer and your rights.
- **Working with Cancer** is an organization which focuses on supporting employers and their employees when someone has cancer. It does however have a lot of free information on its blog www.workingwith-cancer.co.uk.

Writing and journalling

- I run a writing after cancer workshop as part of the **Future Dreams** programme of workshops. Check out the website for more details: www.futuredreams.org.uk.
- *The Artist's Way*, **by Julia Cameron** is an excellent book about how to incorporate journalling into your daily life.

- **The Positive Day Planner** (available from www.thepositivedayplanner.com) is a great little journal with writing prompts, affirmations and places for you to write your gratitude lists.

General resources to help you move on after cancer

- Future Dreams, www.futuredreams.org.uk, provides practical support and advice both on the website and in person at workshops in their London based support centre (most are free but some involve a fee) and are open to people who have completed breast cancer treatment as well as those going through active treatment.
- www.mission-remission.com is a wonderful website which provides an 'interactive platform to share experiences, signpost to relevant services, and advise on practical strategies that help. Through peer support and direct access to research & support services, we aim to make cancer survival less isolating and more empowering, focusing on the positive message that you can feel better after cancer'. They also have a link up with the headspace meditation app which allows you to access Headspace at a reduced cost.
- www.life-aftercancer.co.uk is a London based organization which 'offers a gentle, safe space for you to explore what your life after cancer looks like. We offer individual support through one-to-one coaching, group workshops and support groups, helping you to get from where you are now, to where you want to be. Our spaces are created by trained coaches, all whom have experienced their own personal cancer journey'. Some services are free whilst others incur a charge.
- The wonderful **Younger Breast Cancer Network (YBCN)** on Facebook has a special 'moving on' group that you can join when you finish treatment. Within this (closed, private) group you can chat to other women who are in exactly the same position as you. It is a place to air concerns, worries, questions whilst also providing others with support and sharing stories.
- www.returntowellness.co.uk is the website run by Barbara who has provided her advice in a number of chapters of this book. Her passion is supporting people to manage effectively the emotional impact of a serious health issue, rediscover their purpose and move on with their lives in the way they wish to.

Signs and symptoms of secondary breast cancer

It's important to be aware of the signs and symptoms of secondary breast cancer after you've had primary breast cancer. The secondary breast cancer charity, Make Seconds Count, have produced this helpful

Signs & Symptoms of
Secondary Breast Cancer

Headaches
Ongoing headaches that are not relieved by pain medication.

Vision
Blurred vision, loss of balance or any feeling of weakness and numbness in your arms and legs.

Tiredness
Feeling more tired than usual.

Breathing
Breathlessness and or a persistent dry cough.

Lumps
The discovery of lumps or swollen areas under your arm, in your breast and/or your collarbone areas.

Stomach
Swelling and an uncomfortable feeling in your stomach area.

Pain in bones
Pain in your bones that is not relieved by pain medication. Bone pain may worsen in the evening.

Appetite
Losing your appetite and/or losing weight.

Signs and symptoms of secondary breast cancer will vary in each patient. It is important that you consult a doctor or your local breast cancer clinic if you have any signs or symptoms that:

- Are new or unusual for you
- Do not go away
- Do not have an obvious cause (eg a recent injury or illness)

MAKE
2NDS
COUNT
Giving hope to those affected by
secondary breast cancer

infographic and information to help you understand what to keep an eye on. They have kindly allowed me to reproduce it here. Always, speak to your medical team with any concerns or questions you have.

Signs and symptoms of secondary breast cancer will vary in each patient. It is important that you consult a doctor or your local breast cancer clinic if you have any signs or symptoms that:

- are new or unusual for you;
- do not go away;
- do not have an obvious cause (for example, a recent injury or illness).

Common signs and symptoms:

- Pain in your bones that is not relieved by pain medication – bone pain may worsen in the evening
- breathlessness and or a persistent dry cough
- nausea
- feeling more tired than usual
- ongoing headaches that are not relieved by pain medication
- losing your appetite and/or losing weight
- swelling and an uncomfortable feeling in your stomach area
- blurred vision, loss of balance or any feeling of weakness and numbness in your arms and legs
- the discovery of lumps or swollen areas under your arm, in your breast and/or your collarbone areas

For more information about secondary breast cancer visit www.make2nd-scount.co.uk

Contributors to the book

I'd like to especially thank the wonderful experts for their valuable insight and advice. Thank you for taking the time to talk to me over the course of our many zoom and phone calls, for answering follow-up questions, for reading and checking my written record of your insight and advice, and for generally being so helpful and supportive of this project.

Allie Morgan, Confidence Coach
After being diagnosed with osteosarcoma at the age of 14, Allie always knew that she wanted to provide support to cancer survivors once they finished treatment. While on furlough from her day job in 2020, she completed a Diploma in Life Coaching and became a Certified Confidence Life Coach in order to help survivors get back on their feet after cancer had knocked them down. You can read her confidence tips and find out more at her website www.allie-morgan.com.

Anne Crook, Psycho-Oncology Counsellor Reg MBACP (Accred), BABCP Accred
Anne Crook is an accredited counsellor and psychotherapist with more than 20 years' experience in supporting people affected by cancer. She is the Lead Counsellor with the Psycho-Oncology team at The Christie NHS Foundation Trust, Manchester. Previously, she was the Counsellor for Haemato-Oncology at King's College Hospital, London. Her core training is in psychodynamic psychotherapy and with further training in CBT, she uses a range of therapy approaches to support people at all stages in their treatment and recovery. She regularly contributes to patient groups, events and publications.

Barbara Babcock, Coach and Trainee Family Therapist
Barbara Babcock of Return to Wellness® is a coach and trainee family therapist with over a decade of experience supporting individuals and families to rebuild and renew their lives after a challenging health issue. She has a MA in Coaching Psychology, is a credentialed coach with the International Coaching Federation and has studied Acceptance

Commitment Therapy and Systemic Family Constellations. You can learn more at her website: www.returntowellness.co.uk.

Dr Jane Clark, Consultant Clinical Psychologist BSc (Hons) and ClinPsyD (Doctorate in Clinical Psychology)

Dr Jane Clark qualified as a Clinical Psychologist with a Doctorate in Clinical Psychology from the University of Hull in 2002. During her training, she worked with Professor Leslie Walker at the Oncology drop-in support centres in Hull. Since 2002, Jane has worked at the Leeds Teaching Hospitals NHS Trust in the Department of Clinical and Health Psychology in several clinical specialities. She has worked in the Leeds Cancer Centre since 2004 and is currently a Consultant Clinical Psychologist and lead for the Clinical Psycho-Oncology Team at the Leeds Cancer Centre. Jane's role involves providing psychological assessment and interventions to people going through treatment for cancer, as well as training and supervising other professionals in psychological and communication skills.

Lyndel Moore, Clinical Nurse Lead, Thames Valley Cancer Alliance; Lead Cancer Nurse, Deputy Divisional Director-Head of Cancer Services, The Great Western Hospital Foundation Trust

With many years' experience in senior operational and nursing roles, Lyndel provides professional cancer nursing leadership across work programmes and forms part of the clinical team providing support across cancers services in the Thames Valley Cancer Alliance engaging with trust lead cancer nurses, CAG groups, AHPs and primary care. As Deputy Divisional Director for Cancer Services, Lyndel has led strategic cancer transformation work and supported the Trust in delivery cancer performance resulting in timely treatment for patients using their services with a positive patient experience.

Dr Sophie McGrath, Consultant Medical Oncologist (Breast/Acute Oncology)

Dr Sophie McGrath is a Consultant Medical Oncologist at The Royal Marsden NHS Foundation Trust, specializing in Breast Cancer and Acute Oncology. She studied medicine at Guy's and St Thomas' Hospitals, London, and undertook her oncology training at Imperial College

Healthcare NHS Trust, St George's and Guy's Hospitals, London. She was awarded a PhD from the University of Surrey in 2015, researching biomarkers for early diagnosis, prognosis and treatment response in ovarian cancer. Dr McGrath has worked as a Consultant at The Royal Marsden NHS Foundation Trust and Kingston Hospitals since February 2017, providing compassionate, patient-centred clinical care, to complement her broad experience of chemotherapy, hormonal and targeted therapy, as well as immunotherapy prescribing. Her additional experience as an Acute Oncologist provides a wealth of knowledge around the management of side-effects due to treatment. She has played a pivotal role in the development of the Acute Oncology Service at the Sutton site since 2017.

Endnotes

Introduction

1 These statistics are the ten-year survival rates for 2010 to 2011 as shown on the Cancer Research UK website at the time of writing this book.
2 I realize that this is a miniscule proportion of women who've been through primary breast cancer, and this isn't intended to be any form of research project of a representative sample of women. But it's quite clear that there are enough women who experience certain challenges after completing primary breast cancer, to merit this book.
3 The women who've shared their experiences in this book are all listed at the back of this publication.
4 The experts and professionals are listed at the back of the book in the Contributor section.

Chapter 2

1 The Department of Health and Social Care Report of March 2013, entitled 'Living With and Beyond Cancer: Taking Action to Improve Outcomes'. The report can be found on the UK government website at www.gov.uk/government/publications/living-with-and-beyond-cancer-taking-action-to-improve-outcomes.
2 The insight on Predict in this chapter was provided by Dr Sophie McGrath, Consultant Medical Oncologist at The Royal Marsden NHS Foundation Trust, specializing in Breast Cancer and Acute Oncology.
3 In 2011 the National Cancer Survivorship Initiative carried out some work to understand the needs of those living with cancer and develop models of care that meet their needs. The results of their work can be found here www.ncbi.nlm.nih.gov/pmc/articles/PMC3251952/.

Chapter 3

1 As discussed in Chapter 2, the terminology used at this point differs between hospitals and medics.
2 Remember, as discussed in Chapter 2, follow-ups differ from hospital-to-hospital and depend on the type and extent of cancer you had.

Chapter 4

1 Definition of a psychologist taken from WebMD.com

Chapter 5

1 Dr Jane Clark, Consultant Clinical Psychologist.
2 This analogy is based on ACT – Acceptance and Commitment Therapy.
3 Cancer Research UK https://breastcancernow.org/about-us/media/facts-statistics#develops%20breast%20cancer.
4 Breast Cancer Now https://breastcancernow.org/about-us/media/facts-statistics#develops%20breast%20cancer.

Chapter 6

1 Cancer Research UK https://www.cancerresearchuk.org/health-professional/cancer-statistics/risk/lifetime-risk.

Chapter 8

1 This section on scars was reviewed by Dr Tasha Gandamihardja, Consultant Breast Surgeon.

Chapter 10

1 This chapter provides a general overview of the menopause and hormone therapy and it is important to note that everyone's individual situation is personal to them. Oncologists will consider many factors when prescribing hormone therapy and it is important to speak to your oncologist if you have any questions about your personal situation.
2 This is the average age for a woman to reach menopause but some women will go through it earlier and some later.
3 In addition to acting as a post-treatment hormone therapy, Zoladex has another use. It can be given to women during chemotherapy, as ovarian protection. It can help to preserve ovarian function by putting the ovaries into a state of hibernation preventing the loss of follicles each month. If a woman is on Zoladex for this reason alone, she will stop the treatment after chemotherapy and her periods should return after a few months.
4 See Chapter 2 for more information on the NHS-Predict tool.
5 Rather than referring to 'menopausal symptoms' and 'hormone therapy side-effects' over the course of this chapter, I am going to just use the collective term 'side-effects'.

Chapter 11

1   The terminology surrounding the end of cancer treatment and the status of health of the cancer patient varies from hospital-to-hospital, medic-to-medic and country-to-country. In the UK it is usual for patients to be told that they have 'no evidence of disease', but for people who do not have experience of cancer terminology other than via the media, they may use terms such as 'cured', 'in remission' and 'beaten cancer'.

Chapter 15

1   According to Dr Jane Clark, Consultant Clinical Psychologist.

Chapter 16

1   This is just an example of some of the things that people are told causes cancer.

Chapter 18

1   Thanks to Dr Jane Clark, consultant clinical psychologist, for her advice on post-traumatic growth.

Index